Dear Linda,

Congrats on your little girl. I'm as excited as if she were my own. I hope this book helps with your endeavor of breastfeeding and all the questions that go along with it. I'm here for you!

I love you,
Sonja (& Don too!)

11 2/10/00

BREASTFEEDING

A Holistic Handbook

Also by Eve Adamson

THE COMPLETE IDIOT'S GUIDE TO MASSAGE
(with Joan Budilovsky)
THE COMPLETE IDIOT'S GUIDE TO YOGA
(with Joan Budilovsky)

BREASTFEEDING

A Holistic Handbook

EVE ADAMSON AND MAUREEN KAYS, M.D.

Developed by Amaranth

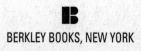

BERKLEY BOOKS, NEW YORK

To our children:
Angus, Emmett, Colleen, Allison, and Andrew

BREASTFEEDING: A HOLISTIC HANDBOOK

This book is an original publication of The Berkley Publishing Group.

A Berkley Book / published by arrangement with
Amaranth

PRINTING HISTORY
Berkley trade paperback edition / January 1999

The Penguin Putnam Inc. World Wide Web site address is
http://www.penguinputnam.com

ISBN: 0-425-16316-4

BERKLEY®
Berkley Books are published by The Berkley Publishing Group,
a member of Penguin Putnam Inc.,
375 Hudson Street, New York, New York 10014.
BERKLEY and the "B" design are trademarks belonging to
Berkley Publishing Corporation.

PRINTED IN THE UNITED STATES OF AMERICA

10 9 8 7 6 5 4 3 2 1

CONTENTS

⚜·INTRODUCTION

*B*Y ITS VERY NATURE, breastfeeding is a holistic practice: body feeding body; mother nurturing baby; touch and nourishment communicating that all is well and safe as your new family provides for your baby's healthy physical, mental, and emotional development. The decision to breastfeed is an intensely personal, intimate, and natural one for both parents. Breastfeeding is not an isolated part of child-rearing. Breastfeeding a baby affects your family's routines and habits in ways you might not expect initially, reaching far into your family's everyday life. How different can it *be* from bottle-feeding, you ask? Very different. A new breastfeeding mother will find herself thinking about her own diet, her level of physical activity, and her ability to deal successfully with stressful situations. After all, the breastfeeding mother is manufacturing her baby's milk with her own body! The commitment to breastfeed your new baby will intimately connect you not only to your baby but to your own body as well: a mother's body beautiful—life-bestowing and life-sustaining. Let us say, however, that breastfeeding is *not* a prerequisite for responsible parenting or successful bonding with your baby. Whatever your new family decides—to breastfeed or not to breastfeed—you will treasure this exciting and precious time with your child forever.

But you think breastfeeding might be right for you? Read on. In this book, new mothers and fathers have a practical, holistic handbook and interactive manual filled with information about all aspects of the breastfeeding experience, presented in a supportive, positive, and easy-to-read format. Most other books we've seen on breastfeeding are either too technical—they read like medical texts—or too limited in scope—they deal with little more than the act of breastfeeding itself and don't give new parents a good idea of what breastfeeding is like when you're doing it day to day. We designed this book to provide a source that tells you everything you *really* need to know about breastfeeding!

Although this book is largely aimed toward the new mother, periodic "Father Alert!" sections give both parents ideas for ways that new fathers can contribute to the breastfeeding experience. He might be nervous or uncomfortable with the idea of breastfeeding, or may not have a clue where he fits in at all, feeling that this is your exclusive territory—off-limits and out-of-bounds. While your partner or spouse's active participation isn't required for you to breastfeed successfully, and some men will be more supportive about breastfeeding than others, we're guessing that he'll be grateful for some strategies that will include him in the process to whatever extent feels right.

This book helps prepare your family for breastfeeding with everything from suggestions for a nursing wardrobe and setting up a nursing haven to tips on teething and knowing when to wean. You will find checklists of what to keep in the diaper bag at all times, how to nurse discreetly in public, ways to make the 2:00 A.M. feeding a pleasure, strategies for handling your feelings of food deprivation, and much, much more. Presented with a holistic approach, one that encompasses all aspects of your family's daily experience, *The Breastfeeding Life* helps your family nurture and sustain the breastfeeding relationship for the entire period you decide to breastfeed your baby.

This book also includes information on such controversial topics as the family bed, breastfeeding while pregnant, breastfeeding your toddler, integrating work and breastfeeding, and breastfeeding an adopted child, presented in a way that will help you to make decisions that are best for your new family. We've even included information addressing the specific needs of women who've undergone breast augmentation or reduction surgery, as well as women who are premenopausal breast cancer survivors and who are eager, in growing numbers, to become pregnant and breastfeed their babies, if possible.

The number of breastfeeding mothers in America is steadily on the rise, with more than half of new mothers giving breastfeeding a try. The U.S. Department of Health and Human Services has set a goal for the year 2000 that 75 percent of women will breastfeed their babies at least through infancy and that 50 percent will continue to breastfeed through the sixth month. The American Academy of Pediatrics currently recommends that all babies be breastfed for at least a full year.

You and your family are about to enter the next stage of the great adventure of life. Ready to start? We wish you, your partner or spouse, your new baby, and your whole family all health and happiness as you begin your journey together. Congratulations!

—Eve Adamson and Maureen Kays, M.D.

Preparing Yourself to Breastfeed

Making the Decision to Breastfeed

BREASTFEEDING is a natural function of the female body, as old as the existence of mammals (after all, *mammal* is defined as an animal whose young feed upon milk from the breast). Indeed, for millennia, breastfeeding was the norm of the human experience. In today's fast-paced world, however, many new families don't believe their lifestyles are necessarily breastfeeding-friendly. Yet bottle-feeding, which only came into vogue in the twentieth century, can be a nuisance of equipment and a constant worry of bacteria and contamination, requiring scrupulous attention to cleansing and sterilization procedures. True, bottle-feeding can also be done at any time, by any person, any place. To many mothers in previous generations, bottle-feeding seemed like a modern miracle—freeing them from the sole responsibility of feeding and enhancing their baby's lives through what was generally thought to be at the time superior advancements in the preparation of formulas that satisfied all a baby's health and nutrition needs. Bottle-feeding also eliminated any discomfort or embarrassment a woman may have felt about breastfeeding.

Some, however, did not agree on the issue of bottle-feeding's advantages. In 1908, J. Ross Snyder wrote in the *Journal of the American Medical Association,* "The deft manipulation of cow's milk to duplicate breast milk is not unlike the claim that by clipping its tail and ears one can so modify the calf that it can be substituted for a baby." Indeed, today's science has revealed the enormous health benefits—to both Mom and her baby—breast-feeding bestows. Scientists now agree with what a lot of people have known all along—Mother Nature really *does* know best.

In the midst of a time of medical breakthroughs and aston-ishing advancements in enhancing and prolonging the human lifespan through technology, researchers have discovered that the primal, natural act of breastfeeding provides the best care and protection for your baby. As more women feel confident about choosing to breastfeed their babies, our society has become more open, encouraging, and supportive of the breastfeeding mother. You *can* include breastfeeding as a vital part of a twenty-first-cen-tury lifestyle. We'll show you how!

Breastfeeding does require commitment, and breastfeeding problems can and often do arise. But then, how many activities in life are problem-free? Many mothers who originally intend to breastfeed sometimes give it up, usually because they aren't fully prepared for what is involved, aren't fully committed to the idea, change their minds, or simply don't know where to turn for help. But virtually all breastfeeding problems can be overcome. We hope you'll agree that the advantages of breastfeeding are well worth the effort. If you decide you want the relationship with your child and family that breastfeeding fosters, commit and stay with it! Be sure the pediatrician you choose is a strong supporter of breastfeeding, then don't let anyone dissuade you. Summon support from inside yourself—from your brain, which knows breastfeeding is best, and from your heart, which feels how right it is. If you are already breastfeeding as you read this book, hang in there! You are eager to get as much information as you can and you've come to the right place. Use this chapter to take a look at some of the specific benefits of breastfeeding for your new family.

WHAT BREASTFEEDING MEANS FOR YOUR BABY

The image of breastfeeding throughout history has been one of the power and mystical life-sustaining force of the mother's breast. The breastfeeding mother is an important cultural symbol and the way a society perceives her can speak volumes. In our own country, research psychologists are continually discovering fresh evidence to support the theory that a child's first connections and life experiences directly impact the nature of her personality throughout life. Breastfeeding, then, can be one of the most important early connections between mother and child. In addition to the profound health and immune system benefits breastfeeding affords your infant, the new family's breastfeeding relationship is life-affirming for the baby in every other sense. Breastfeeding promotes an intimate and essential bond, both physical and emotional, between mother and baby. Breastfeeding gives your baby the best possible nourishing and nurturing.

The Nurturing Bond

An infant has relatively few effective communication skills. Your baby has intense needs and wants, but cannot easily express them for caregivers. How frustrating! There is one language your baby can understand fluently, however: the first language, the language of feeding. Hunger, the need to suck, the need to be touched and held close to a mother's body are all primary, fierce needs that are consummately fulfilled when you breastfeed your baby.

Breastfeeding communicates what your baby can't yet understand verbally: your love, your affection, your touch, her safety, and the complete fulfillment of those remarkably profound needs. The skin-to-skin contact your baby experiences with you is how nature intended her to be fed. Of course, if you bottle-feed, your baby can still receive nourishment, touch, and bonding from you. Bottle-fed babies are also held close and nurtured

4 · Breastfeeding: A Holistic Handbook

by their mothers, and these babies thrive as well. However, formula fortified with supplements fed from a latex nipple heated by an artificial heat source can only imitate what nature does best and, well, . . . *naturally.* (And, by the way, *for free!*) Your baby *wants* to breastfeed. Instinct draws her irresistibly to your breast, and your body has prepared itself throughout your pregnancy to feed her. Fulfilling her nutritive needs this way is a beautifully natural thing to do.

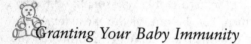

Granting Your Baby Immunity

The power of breastmilk to protect your baby from illness is awe-inspiring. Breastmilk provides him with immunity throughout the entire course of lactation, even into the toddler years, as long as you continue to nurse. Breastfed babies commonly experience fewer upper respiratory infections, ear infections (otitis media), episodes of diarrhea, and allergic reactions.

Simply, here's how it works:

Unlike artificial milk (formula), breastmilk is teeming with living cells, called leukocytes (white blood cells): neutrophils kill bacteria on the body's internal surfaces and macrophages penetrate tissue, helping to maintain stomach and intestinal protection for the first four to five months of your baby's life. These leukocytes kill disease-causing organisms with extraordinary vehemence. In fact, a couple of drops of breastmilk up your baby's nose or in his ear will kill bacteria there, too! Even frozen breastmilk will retain its immunity boosters (although heating in a microwave will destroy the macrophages). Formula, of course, contains none of these components—and even though a new formula has recently been developed that contains added nucleotides (the building blocks of genes) that seem to offer some added protection, research still clearly demonstrates breastmilk's superior and inimitable immune-boosting properties.

Colostrum, the yellowish to clear, thick, supernutritious fluid your body makes for your baby in the first few days after birth, before your mature milk comes in, protects from many diseases to which infants might otherwise be susceptible with their under-developed immune systems, including polio, staphylococcus, and many other dangerous diseases. Colostrum contains less fat and more protein than the breastmilk that comes later. Even if you only breastfeed for one week, your baby will be significantly more protected than a formula-fed baby, due to the potent effects of colostrum. In fact, the best thing you can do for your baby's health is to expose her to colostrum.

Secretory immunoglobulin A is the secret to human milk's immunity protection. Known as IgA, this compound is generated in the mammary glands and protects against molecules that might cause allergic reactions in your baby; it also provides antibodies helpful in preventing infant diarrhea and certain respiratory problems. The IgA antibodies prevent pathogens (disease-producing bacteria or microorganisms) from attaching themselves to the digestive or respiratory tracts. By breastfeeding, you are providing your baby with antibodies to whatever pathogens you have encountered. Even if you catch a cold or flu virus while breast-feeding, you will quickly develop antibodies to that virus that will be secreted in your milk almost before you start showing symptoms! If your baby catches that cold, he'll be much less likely to suffer complications such as pneumonia or otitis media (ear infections). Unfortunately, this only applies to germs to which you have actually been exposed. He can still catch colds and other contagious conditions from other people, most notoriously other children in daycare, or from big brother or sister in daycare or school. Keep in mind that the antibodies you provide through your milk are really just "lent" to your baby, and won't trigger his own production of those antibodies. Therefore, this protection lasts only as long as you are nursing. The longer you nurse, though, the more time you give that young and inexperienced immune system to build up its own personal store of antibodies.

If you or your partner or spouse tend to suffer from allergies,

GOOD STUFF IN BREASTMILK

Protein: Protein in mother's milk is specifically formulated to grow a human baby. Cow's milk has far too much protein, and is, of course, meant to grow a baby cow.

Fat and cholesterol: On average, about 40 percent of the calories in mother's milk comes from fat (fat content in your milk varies throughout the first year, over the course of a day, even from beginning to end of a single feeding). Babies need fat and cholesterol, too. The high cholesterol content in mother's milk may prepare a baby's system for handling cholesterol as an adult. It is also responsible for the development of nerve coverings. The human brain contains a lot of cholesterol, and evidence suggests that the cholesterol in human breastmilk facilitates babies' brain growth.

Lysozyme: An antibacterial enzyme, also present in saliva and tears, that dissolves the cell walls of harmful bacteria, soothes inflamed tissue, and acts as a disinfectant in eyes, noses, mammary glands, and throughout the nursing baby's digestive system. Lysozyme can be added to formula, but it is destroyed by the sterilization process.

Lactoferrin: This protein makes up approximately one-third of the protein in human milk (cow's milk is primarily casein). Lactoferrin is much more digestible than casein and also absorbs iron molecules. Many pathogens, like *E. coli*, need iron molecules to metabolize, but with lactoferrin present, the pathogens have a slimmer chance of being able to flourish.

Oligosaccharides: These human milk sugars fight disease-causing organisms in much the same way antibodies do.

Antioxidants: These substances act as anti-inflammatory agents in a baby's digestive tract, deterring the pain and inflammation that can be a natural side-effect of the body's efforts to fight disease.

Lactose: This human milk sugar helps to maintain babies' intestinal flora, in addition to providing calories and a pleasantly sweet taste. Some children and adults develop an intolerance for lactose in cow's milk, but the lactose in human breastmilk is tailor-made for babies and intolerance is rare.

Lots of vitamins and minerals: All a baby needs for the first six months of life, conveniently provided in perfect dosages, even when what you are eating is less than perfect.

Lots of enzymes, hormones, peptides, and other goodies: Science has yet to fully understand and determine all the components of human milk, but so far we haven't been able to develop a formula that equals it. The constitution of human breastmilk is the product of centuries of evolution, nature's working scientist.

your baby will be more susceptible, but breastfeeding can help by contributing a variety of compounds to his system to help fight allergic reactions. Postponing the introduction of any solid foods may be your best weapon against food allergy. The baby with a propensity toward food allergies may be able to remain reaction-free by subsisting solely on breastmilk through the sixth month or slightly beyond. Exposure to particularly complex proteins (such as those found in cow's milk and eggs) can cause allergic reactions in a baby whose immature digestive system isn't ready for the job. Even excessive cow's milk consumption by you can trigger an allergic reaction in your breastfeeding infant who may handle the same substances just fine if introduction to these foods is delayed. (But don't let that stop you from enjoying two to four cups of milk each day while nursing.)

Breastfeeding isn't just good for baby. It serves Mom well, too. Let's start with the hormone prolactin. The act of breastfeeding releases prolactin into your bloodstream, which has the effect of stimulating a maternal impulse. If you are worried about whether you will ever be "the maternal type," we can assure you that your body's natural production of prolactin will bring out your mothering feelings. The hormone also has a relaxing effect, which compels you to sit down and take time out so you can get the most from breastfeeding during the day. For those of you who are always on the run, prolactin helps you take down the pace and use feeding times to rest and revitalize.

Emotions and maternal instincts aside, when you breastfeed you get to eat five hundred extra calories every day and not gain any extra weight! Remember that extra fat you accumulated during pregnancy (how could you forget!)? It was all for this. In fact, as long as you don't gorge yourself every day, breastfeeding itself should melt away all that extra weight almost effortlessly over the course of the first year (for some, even sooner).

After you spend a few weeks getting the hang of it, breastfeeding is simplicity itself. When you breastfeed, the baby's food is always conveniently at hand, premixed, presterilized, and at the perfect temperature. Your breasts will produce as much milk as your baby needs. Your baby will reward you, too, with dirty diapers that are far more pleasant to change (and to smell) than the diapers of formula-fed babies.

Breastfeeding will help your uterus contract faster and return to its prepregnancy shape. You'll experience less postpartum bleeding, too. This happens through the action of a hormone, called oxytocin, which is released by the pituitary gland when breastfeeding begins. Although the verdict is still out regarding whether breastfeeding reduces your risk of breast cancer, many compelling studies strongly suggest a correlation, especially for premenopausal breast cancer. Breast cancer rates

YOU CAN GO FROM BREASTFEEDING TO BOTTLE-FEEDING, BUT NOT (USUALLY) FROM BOTTLE-FEEDING TO BREASTFEEDING

If you start out bottle-feeding and then change your mind and want to breastfeed, it may be quite difficult, sometimes impossible, to start producing milk after you have signaled your body to stop by not breastfeeding in the first days. If you start out breastfeeding and establish a good milk supply, you can always decide to stop later. Breastfeeding in the hospital or birthing center right after delivery and in the early weeks at home gives you more options. It also exposes your baby to colostrum, the potent and highly beneficial fluid your breasts produce in the first few days postpartum. And you're taking advantage of an opportunity to enhance your early physical bond with your baby in her first important days of life.

are low to nonexistent in many cultures where bottle-feeding is low to nonexistent, while in the United States, where bottle-feeding is fairly common, breast cancer, too, is common. Extended breastfeeding (longer than one year) may lower your risk even further. (Research also suggests that if your mother breastfed you, your risk may be reduced yet again!) There is also some evidence that breastfeeding can help prevent or lessen the effects of osteoporosis.

Because breastfeeding tends to suppress ovulation, you may think you won't have to worry about getting pregnant again as long as you are breastfeeding. Don't depend on this! We know more than a few women who "risked it just once" and were pregnant again when their babies were just a few months old. If you shouldn't or don't want to get pregnant again right away, consult your physician to choose a form of safe and reliable birth control. Also, menstruation often stays away as long as you are breast-feeding, and studies have shown that this suppressed ovulation during pregnancy and breastfeeding may help protect you against the threat of ovarian cancer.

Lastly, engorged postpartum breasts will give you a fullness you've never experienced before. True, pregnancy may have given you some stretch marks and a little less buoyancy to your once jaunty breasts, but if you weren't generously endowed prepregnancy, now your postpartum engorged breasts are filling out the tops of your clothes like never before. Once you've been nursing for a while, your breasts will gradually return to their normal size, although some women remain bigger breasted than before. (If you are already full breasted, worry not—the larger you are to begin with, the less your breast size is likely to increase during pregnancy and lactation.)

How Your Body Prepares for Breastfeeding

Toward the end of your pregnancy, the body you remember is just a shadow of your new, prodigious self. Your breasts, too, are probably becoming larger than they were, and as early as your sixth month of pregnancy, you may notice colostrum leaking from your breasts, or you may be able to express it by gently squeezing at the base of your nipple area. While your body is diligently sustaining your baby and preparing itself for labor, your breasts are busy with a different task: preparing to nourish your baby once she is out here with the rest of us. This is no small task, and the production of milk is an amazing process.

Deep inside your breast, small glands called alveoli produce milk. These glands are surrounded by special cells that squeeze the milk into ducts. The milk then moves into enlarged tubes called lactiferous sinuses. When your baby nurses, she first drains the lactiferous sinuses, which serve as a sort of "holding tank" for milk that is immediately available. You will feel the tingling of the milk ejection reflex, also called "letdown," as the cells surrounding the alveoli contract, squeezing milk from these glands and surrounding ducts toward the nipple. This "hindmilk" is richer and thicker than the first milk, or "foremilk." Your baby should take the entire areola (the brown area around the nipple) in her mouth, not just the nipple, to drain the lactiferous sinuses and extract the rich hindmilk from the ducts and alveoli. If your baby latches onto the nipple only, you'll also be more likely to experience nipple soreness.

THROUGHOUT YOUR PREGNANCY

During the first trimester of pregnancy, months one through three, the ducts in your breast begin to multiply and the small bumps on your areola called Montgomery glands increase in size, appearing like small pimples. The skin of the areola and the nipple darken and the Montgomery glands on the areola begin to produce a lubricant that kills bacteria and keeps your nipples sterile (this is why you don't need to wash your nipples with soap, and why your breasts can't become contaminated by touching—the glands will do their job as long as you are nursing). All these developments will make your breasts tender and sore, one of the first signs of pregnancy for many women.

In the second trimester, months four through six, the ducts continue to multiply and the alveoli begin to produce colostrum, the clear to yellowish fluid that will nourish your baby before your milk comes in. Your breasts now become noticeably larger and heavier with the increased tissue and fluid. Even if your baby is born prematurely at the end of the second trimester, your breasts will produce sufficient colostrum to nourish him.

You might get stretch marks in your third trimester, months six through nine, the result of heredity and/or skin

FATHER ALERT!

BREASTFEEDING BENEFITS FOR NEW FATHERS

Here are some breastfeeding plusses you fathers might want to consider:

◉ Let's be frank: if Mom is breastfeeding, you aren't going to have to learn to prepare formula (though you may want to help out occasionally by feeding your baby expressed breastmilk in a bottle).

◉ If you've become the sole financial support for your family through the mutual decision that your partner or spouse will stay home, temporarily or indefinitely, with your baby, you may be worried about making ends meet. Do you know how expensive formula is? You don't want to know. Add to that bottles, rings, nipples, bottle warmers, sterilizers . . .

◉ Your baby is forming an intense emotional bond with his mother at this early developmental stage. Research confirms that breastfeeding will help to make him secure and well-adjusted, which means that his relationship with you will be healthier and happier, especially in the toddler years when he is less dependent on Mom and begins to imitate (and idolize!) you.

◉ Breastfed babies mean lower doctor's bills. A 1994–95 study by Kaiser-Permanente (a large health maintenance organization, or HMO) showed that infants breastfed for at least six months had $1,435 less in health care claims in 1993 than infants who were formula-fed! In fact, a 1994 study conducted by Johns Hopkins University revealed that out of a sample of eighty-nine fathers of bottle-feeding newborns, less than one-third had any idea that breastfed babies were at a lower risk for disease than bottle-fed babies. See how enlightened you've become?

stretched by so much additional weight. These often disappear sometime in the first year after the birth, or become much less noticeable as your breasts and skin shrink back to normal. Third trimester breast size is approximately postpartum breast size, so you can buy nursing bras now, but allow a little room, particularly for the engorged breasts of the first few weeks. (See "Your Nursing Wardrobe," page 26.) If you want to try nipple preparation, this is the time. Most women's nipples are protruding by the third trimester, but if yours are inverted, you and your partner can begin to practice some of the techniques, outlined in the next few pages, that are designed to correct inverted nipples.

During the entire pregnancy, while your breasts are preparing for milk production, your body is increasing its levels of prolactin. After these nine months, prolactin, estrogen, and progesterone levels in your body are all high. However, after the placenta is delivered, your levels of estrogen and progesterone drop sharply, which signals your alveoli to begin official milk production. This will happen no matter what sort of delivery you experienced, vaginal or cesarean. Once the "begin production" signal has been given, every time you nurse your baby, your levels of prolactin soar and your body increases milk production. The more you nurse, the more milk you will produce. The system is perfect. Your body will make just as much milk as your baby needs for as long as you continue to nurse regularly.

BREAST TERMINOLOGY
Know your breast! Impress your physician!

Alveoli: Small, sacklike glands that manufacture milk deep inside your breast.

Areola: The darkened area of skin surrounding the nipple.

Colostrum: The clear to yellowish substance your breasts provide for the first few days after birth, before your milk comes in; nutrient-rich and full of antibodies, colostrum is extremely beneficial to your newborn.

Ducts: Small tubes that allow passage of the milk from the alveoli to the nipple openings.

Foremilk: The milk stored in the breasts' lactiferous sinuses; typically thinner, lighter in color, and less caloric than the hindmilk, to encourage continued feeding.

Hindmilk: The milk at the end of the feeding; thicker, whiter, and more caloric, signaling baby that he is satiated.

Lactiferous sinuses: Wider areas at the ends of the ducts in which foremilk pools, ready for baby's sucking to extract it.

Letdown: Another name for the milk ejection reflex.

Lobules: Grapelike clusters of alveoli.

Montgomery glands: Small, pimple-like glands on the areola that secrete a substance that maintains nipple sterility. Also called Montogomery's tubercle.

Oxytocin: The hormone responsible for the milk ejection reflex, which signals cells surrounding ducts to contract and move the milk through the ducts to the nipple. It also induces the uterus to contract faster after delivery.

Prolactin: The hormone that signals milk production and other beneficial maternal processes and feelings.

Protractility: The ability of the nipple to protrude.

PREPARING YOUR BREASTS DURING PREGNANCY

Actually, there is no hard evidence that any type of breast preparation will alleviate future nipple soreness. However, pregnancy is a good time to become more familiar with your breasts, particularly if you aren't used to paying any special attention to them. Look at your breasts in the mirror. Touch them. Feel how heavy each breast has become. Look for leaking colostrum. It isn't a good idea to get in the habit of expressing colostrum during pregnancy (although expressing a few drops occasionally won't hurt, just to get the feel of it and to see what it looks like). Researchers aren't sure whether the breast produces a fixed amount of colostrum or whether colostrum is continually manufactured in the breast. Also, evidence exists that shows that *extensive* nipple stimulation can induce premature labor, but don't let this scare you away from your breasts. By extensive, we mean for several hours every day.

If you do want to prepare your nipples, there are some things you can do during the third trimester, including exposing your nipples to the air and sunlight (try not to shock the neighbors), pressing your nipples lightly with a towel when you dry off after a shower (avoid heavy friction, which can unnecessarily dry the skin), wearing bras and clothing made of natural, breathable fabric (stay away from tight sports bras or underwire bras that can decrease circulation), and letting your partner or spouse touch and rub your nipples. Try gentle tugging, rolling the nipples between your fingers, and generally getting them accustomed to touch. Gentle breast massage is great, too, and very relaxing if your partner does it and you are comfortable with it. The more your breasts are touched, the more easy you will be with the touching. Don't do anything that hurts or is uncomfortable in any way, however. Rubbing nipples briskly or handling breasts roughly should be avoided.

Using soap or lotion on your nipples is unnecessary and undesirable. Your breasts' own Montgomery glands keep the nipples clean, and you don't want to clog the pores and infect the ducts. During the third trimester and especially in the first few days postpartum, however, you will have access to the perfect natural lubricant: colostrum! If colostrum has leaked from your breast or you have expressed a little, rub it into the nipple. This will keep the skin moist and conditioned without clogging the pores. If your breasts are very dry, you may also use a few drops of vegetable oil.

Some women have inverted nipples, and this condition isn't anything to worry about. Inverted nipples usually correct themselves by the third trimester. If they haven't, however, you will want to draw them out so your baby can breastfeed more easily. Have your doctor examine your breasts, then ask your doctor to offer suggestions about correcting nipple inversion (usually an easy process). Your doctor may suggest wearing breast shells, which press on the base of the nipples, encouraging each to protrude through an openings in the middle, or he or she may suggest techniques for gently pressing or pulling the base of the nipple, or regularly pulling the nipple out and rolling it between your fingers. Keep trying, and please don't think that inverted nipples mean you can't breastfeed. Your breasts *will* respond with a little encouragement.

FINDING SUPPORT AND INFORMATION ABOUT BREASTFEEDING

In almost every case where breastfeeding is unsuccessful, lack of information and support is the culprit. In the past, many women

FATHER ALERT!

NEW FATHERS CAN HELP, TOO
(It's More Fun than Changing Diapers!)

Breastfeeding success depends on many things, not the least of which is expectant parents becoming familiar and comfortable with Mom's breasts. Maybe you have always thought of them as "yours." This isn't uncommon. You know, of course, that their primary function is to nurse a baby, though . . . don't you? That doesn't mean you won't ever be able to touch them again, however. In fact, during the last trimester of pregnancy, you can help your partner prepare to breastfeed your new baby by helping her become comfortable with her breasts. Learn the gentle art of breast massage, and the skill could come in handy for years to come. Show an interest in your partner's changing, growing breasts. If you are interested rather than put off by such things as leaking colostrum and feeling for the milk ducts, not only will she grow more comfortable with her body and sharing it with you, but she will be infinitely reassured that breastfeeding will succeed. Be lighthearted about the entire affair. (After the baby comes, you may discover that milk-shooting breasts can be fun!)

worried that they couldn't produce milk, that their breasts were too big or too small, or that their breastmilk wouldn't be rich enough. These fears persist in many women even today. In addition, some women feel they may be unlikely candidates for breastfeeding because they work and their careers will make breastfeeding a logistical nightmare, or that because of a cesarean section or for other health reasons, breastfeeding is not an option for their new families Today, virtually all of these "problems" are

It's All in the Family

In our grandmothers' and great-grandmothers' days, women passed on the art of breastfeeding from generation to generation. Granted, breastfeeding occurred behind closed doors in those days, in the privacy of the home and, most likely, out of view of anyone, with grandmother and other female relatives as occasional supervisors and confidantes. However, these women had the advantage of reliable access to a time-honored tradition of breastfeeding knowledge. Unfortunately, it is all too common that a woman who chooses to breastfeed today will not have the benefit of her own mother's breastfeeding experiences to draw upon. Historically speaking, this is unusual! By the early 1970s, bottle-feeding had become so popular that only one in four women breastfed their babies—an all-time low that has since turned around. If your mother breastfed you in those days, she was considered progressive indeed, and no doubt she'll be a great source of comfort and wisdom for you. A breastfeeding mother we know told us that her own mother had a very difficult time in the '70s convincing the nurses and doctor at the hospital where she delivered to allow her to breastfeed. "You don't need to bother with that," they told her mother. "We can take care of everything for you. Just rest and relax." This woman, now a grandmother in the 1990s, insisted on breastfeeding and can look back with pride on having followed her instincts.

But even if she didn't breastfeed you or your brothers and sisters, encourage your mother to understand your own interest in breastfeeding and to help you learn everything about it. You may find that your mother is as eager, curious, and excited about breastfeeding as you are. She may not be able to give you that invaluable tip about what to do if your baby obviously prefers feeding from one breast over another (see page 52 for the answer) or what to do about a nasty

case of thrush (see page 153 for the answer)—you might
have to turn to a friend from your breastfeeding support
group for that information—but she'll be there to offer you
encouragement, love, and, if you're lucky, baby-sitting services, anytime you need them.

not considered serious impediments to breastfeeding and there
are effective strategies to deal with them.

With proper education, instruction, and practice, nearly all
women can breastfeed if they *choose* to breastfeed. Breastfeeding
is difficult—*at first!* Don't be afraid to ask for help! If you stay
committed to the breastfeeding life, you will be successful.
Appendix B, "Resources," at the back of this book, lists numer-
ous organizations, books, and on-line references and forums that
may prove invaluable as you find out more about breastfeeding
and prepare for the delivery of your baby. Generally, a couple of
weeks are all it takes to become a master.

The most important thing to remember is this: fear and lack
of confidence are the common results of misinformation and poor
communication. If you are interested in breastfeeding, ask your
physician about local support groups of breastfeeding mothers.
(Or call the La Leche League International in Illinois at 312-455-
7730 between 9:00 A.M. and 3:00 P.M. Central Time for information about groups in your area.) Join a support group while you
are still pregnant and get the benefit of other mothers' experiences
and encouragement before you begin. If you are already breastfeeding your baby and are reading this book because you are having difficulty finding good sources of support and information, a
community group of breastfeeding mothers can help you, too.
Even an expectant or new father can benefit. If the man you love
is supportive but feels awkward and maybe even a little afraid of
the breastfeeding process, ask if he can talk to the partners or
spouses of some of the women in your group about *their* feelings

and experiences about their partners' choices to breastfeed—that is, of course, if he is open to the idea. With a little coaxing from you, he may agree to try expressing his thoughts and concerns with other men who're going through it. A father who is reluctant about breastfeeding often ends up enchanted with his breastfeeding family. Give him time. On the other hand, he might be your biggest champion of the breastfeeding life from the get go!

Don't be shy about asking health care professionals any questions you might have. It's their job to help you! Set up home visits from a certified lactation consultant, someone who is specially trained in breastfeeding techniques, for after your delivery; you can reach these consultants through the hospital where you deliver(ed) or through your pediatrician. In many hospitals and birthing centers, you'll automatically be visited by a lactation consultant if you plan to breastfeed. Plan for additional support by asking friends who've breastfed their children to visit you in the first few weeks postpartum to answer questions and offer advice and encouragement. And of course, there's always *your* mom, who can be an invaluable source of information if she breastfed you, and even if she didn't! (She may wish she had.)

If you try breastfeeding and decide to stop for any reason along the way, *don't feel guilty!* New mothers have enough sources of stress. Know that you'll feel good about the time and effort you've spent to give your baby the benefits of breastfeeding that you've just read about, and that you'll cherish the breastfeeding haven you shared together. In the meantime, give in to your present enthusiasm and curiosity. Continue to explore what breastfeeding means to you and to your new family.

2

Preparing Your Home for Breastfeeding

Nesting: Making Your Home Nursing Friendly

In the last trimester of pregnancy, you will have probably cut back, at least to some extent, on your usual activities. Now is your time to "nest," to prepare your home for its new occupant, to get into that maternal state of mind. You can do several things at this stage to make breastfeeding a lot easier in the first weeks postpartum.

Three areas of your home that will need your attention are the kitchen, your wardrobe closet, and the place where you will nurse your baby. Clearly, nutrition is a primary concern of the nursing mother and you'll want to be eating right when you bring your baby home. Even with help from your partner or spouse, your mother, friends, or part-time caregivers, cooking may be a challenge. Advance planning will ensure that you and your new baby will have the benefits of a healthy diet—and not have to worry about who's cooking!

Just as with anything else in life, having the right clothing and accessories can mean the difference between comfort and discomfort, success and failure with breastfeeding.

You wouldn't normally wear a sports bra to a cocktail party (then again, maybe an adventurous woman might!) or high heels when you're about to run a marathon; neither will you want to wear uncomfortable or inappropriate clothes while breastfeeding. We'll fill you in on what's comfortable to wear and convenient to have on hand.

The most important place to consider when preparing your home for breastfeeding is your nursing haven. The right nursing haven for you will have a lot to do with your lifestyle and personal preferences. We'll help you design a nursing haven that suits your personality and enhances your baby's comfort.

You'll also want to consider your breastfeeding needs when you begin to think about family sleeping arrangements, which will directly affect everyone's—mother's, father's, and baby's— experience of nighttime feedings. Yes, a good night's sleep *is* possible when you are breastfeeding! And while you're at it, take a look around the whole house with an eye toward creating a safe, natural environment for your new family.

You're Still Eating for Two

You can't even imagine how much you won't want to cook when you first get home from the hospital. One of the kindest things you can do for yourself in those last few weeks of pregnancy (assuming you don't deliver early) is to prepare about a week's worth of meals that can be frozen and easily reheated. You will be recovering and your body will need good, healthy good—not fast food junk or frozen dinners! You will probably end up ordering take-out a few times (look for healthy take-out choices) and Dad and other family members can pitch in, too; but on those first few evenings, everyone will be exhausted and an effortless, home-cooked meal could be just the remedy everyone needs to feel good again.

Cook a whole turkey or chicken. Slice the meat, and put it in freezer bags. Make mashed potatoes (easy to make from scratch, which is so much more nutritious than instant), mound individual portions on a cookie sheet, freeze, then remove frozen mounds and store in a large freezer bag. Store the meat, potatoes, and a box of frozen broccoli, green beans, or other favorite vegetables together in the freezer (a basket is good for this purpose). When you are ready to have the meal, arrange the meat in the middle of a roasting pan surrounded by the mashed potato mounds, and heat in a 350-degree oven for thirty minutes or until the meat is hot. Meanwhile, cook the vegetables in the microwave.

Homemade lasagna freezes beautifully right in the baking pan (try veggie lasagna with spinach noodles for a nutritious change of pace), as does homemade macaroni and cheese. Whoever isn't watching the baby can mix a quick salad and you have a wonderful meal. A purchased loaf of French or Italian bread, brushed with olive oil and spread with fresh garlic put through a garlic press, then broiled for a few minutes, makes an elegant accompaniment. Experiment with freezing your family's favorite casseroles, or try some of the recipes in the Mini Family Cookbook that begins on page 245—for example, the "Hearty Spaghetti Casserole" or "Freezable French Toast Brunch."

You will also want to stock the refrigerator and pantry with easy-to-eat items such as prewashed baby carrots (a wonderfully healthful snack for nursing mothers), whole wheat crackers, peanut butter (the natural kind without sugar is best), dried fruit, nuts, cereal (preferably the varieties low in sugar, high in fiber, with added iron), yogurt, apples, citrus fruits, other seasonal fruits, bagels, hard-boiled eggs, cheese, milk, and lots of juice. Fill your freezer with cans of frozen apple, cranberry, calcium-added orange, and other juice concentrates (look for varieties that are 100 percent juice; avoid varieties that list high-fructose corn syrup as an ingredient). Staying hydrated while nursing is essential; a good stock of juices gives mother and baby a selection of

FATHER ALERT!

IF YOU DON'T COOK, IT'S TIME TO LEARN

We apologize ahead of time to all you men who share the cooking duties, and especially to those of you who are the exclusive family cooks. However, many men still don't cook—and you know who you are! Even before your baby has joined your family, you may want to make an effort to get into the habit of helping in the kitchen. A woman in her third trimester of pregnancy (not to mention a nauseated woman in her first trimester) probably won't be too fired up about cooking. Help her by asking what you can do, offer to take over completely, or simply put the food away after the meal and wash the dishes.

When your baby finally does make his appearance and your partner is nursing, she'll need your help more than ever. Needless to say, she has a lot on her mind besides cooking family dinners, and you will be doing her a great service if you handle kitchen duty, especially for the first few weeks. Who knows—you may never let your partner back in the kitchen again! Look in the Mini Family Cookbook at the back of this book for cooking hints especially for new fathers.

nutrients and mother (for purely selfish reasons!) a little variety in taste sensation. A quick whirl in the blender eliminates the need for perpetual stirring and makes the juice taste almost creamy. Having these foods ready in your refrigerator when you come home from the hospital can be a lifesaver when you are starving, the baby is crying, and you are too exhausted even to look for a cooking utensil.

YOUR NURSING WARDROBE

Mothers living the breastfeeding life must dress for the occasion, but not all maternity clothes are nursing friendly—and you're sick of those tent dresses, anyway. Rather than being caught without a thing to wear when you first decide to venture out on an errand or a social call, be prepared by assembling a nursing wardrobe before you go into labor. A functional nursing wardrobe needn't be expensive. You probably have many, if not all, of the basics already.

The most important concept for your nursing wardrobe is *access*. Your baby needs frequent access to you, while you need to feel comfortable and unexposed. First and foremost, you'll want a selection of nursing bras, a brilliant invention that allows you to lower a front flap with one hand, while still maintaining the support and cover of a bra. You'll want to wait until your eighth month of pregnancy to purchase a nursing bra, because throughout your pregnancy your breasts will continue to grow and you won't know your true nursing size until this time. Then, allow a little room because especially in the first few weeks, you will frequently be engorged, which swells the breasts even more.

Try on different brands of nursing bras. Practice fastening and unfastening the flaps so you can find a style comfortable on you and that you feel is easy to manipulate. You'll want at least three nursing bras, more if you can afford it (good nursing bras aren't cheap), because when your milk comes in, you'll leak and bras will pile up in the laundry basket faster than you can wash them. Also, invest in some nursing pads. These cloth or disposable pads look like small round shoulder pads or sanitary napkins. You wear them inside your bra to prevent leaking onto bras and clothing. Sometimes even thinking about your baby or hearing her cry will result in the milk ejection reflex, and if you are out in public, it can be embarrassing to leak through your shirt. Also try wearing prints as a good way to camouflage if you leak or accidentally

Your Nursing Wardrobe

The longer you nurse, the better you will fit into your prepregnancy clothes and the less you will need to worry about leakage, but the following list is a great wardrobe to launch your nursing career:

◉ Three to five good nursing bras.

◉ At least two loose dresses with button-down fronts.

◉ At least four button-down blouses.

◉ At least four large, baggy or trapeze-style tops (maternity tops work well).

◉ Two or three pairs of leggings and several pairs of comfortable shorts or long pants (depending on the season).

◉ Washable nursing pads—as many as you can afford! (The disposable kind are handy, too.)

get milk on your clothing. After you've been nursing for a few months, you won't have to worry about leaking anymore.

If you really don't want to purchase a nursing bra, you may find that a regular bra can be pushed aside or lifted up or down to facilitate nursing. If you are more comfortable doing this, by all means, go ahead and try it. Also, particularly if you are relatively small-breasted, you may be able to get away with going braless, at least when you are at home, and especially after the first few months of nursing when your breasts start to get back to normal. Many nursing mothers abandon their bras while at home because it is more comfortable and provides quicker access for the baby. It probably won't make you any "saggier," and you don't have to worry about exposure in the privacy of your own home, so you might as well be comfortable. The important thing is to find what works for you. There is no right or wrong way.

If you are a sports bra aficionado, you may need to lay them aside for a while. While they offer great support, they aren't usually cut for the nursing mother's full size, and even those that fit tend to be tight, which can trigger leakage and cut off circulation, as well as making access difficult. Only full-cut sports bras that open in front and aren't too tight are a possibility for nursing if you simply aren't ready to try anything else.

Now for your outerwear. Some maternity shops and specialty catalogues sell clothes designed specifically for nursing, but most of them are more functional than attractive, to be honest. If you can find something you like, great. However, there are other options. Loose dresses and shirts with buttons down the front are flexible and comfortable. Simply unbutton as far as necessary, and dinner is served! Or, unbutton from the bottom instead of the top for more discreet nursing and more warmth for the baby. Look for clothes with relatively large buttons that aren't too difficult to undo. A beautiful dress with fifty tiny buttons isn't very practical. A comfortable jumper with four large buttons over a T-shirt is perfect because you can unbutton, lift up the T-shirt, and still have the top of your chest covered (and warm—if it's winter, you'll be thankful). You can also cut slits in an old T-shirt to wear under loose sweaters or jumpers. Put the shirt on and mark the slits a few inches over each nipple before you cut.

You'll also want a selection of large, baggy, trapeze-style shirts (the kind that expand out towards the hem in an A shape). You probably have some of these from your maternity wardrobe. Don't pack them away just yet. They are comfortable, flattering, they probably still fit better than your prepregnancy shirts, and they make a perfect tent to drape over a nursing baby in public. Paired with leggings, large shirts are a great way to nurse discreetly. Once baby is under there, no one can catch a glimpse of anything, and he can get an often much-needed break from the

THE SLING:
A NURSING MOTHER'S SAVIOR

One of the great inventions for nursing mothers and babies is based on a concept familiar to ancient cultures all over the world (TV's frontier doctor Michaela "Mike" Quinn used one while nursing TV baby Katie—a gift from Native Americans). The sling is a long piece of fabric draped and sewn to hold your baby against your chest. Such a position is comforting to her and convenient for you if you are running errands, working at your computer, doing housework, or engaging in anything else that demands the use of your hands. A few minor manipulations of clothing and your nursing bra, and she can nurse while you go virtually hands-free! In the first few months, she will thrive best if she is with you, on you, being held against you absolutely as much as possible. The sling makes this easy, convenient, and fun.

A variety of slings and infant carriers are on the market. Infant carriers are like small backpacks you wear on your front, in which your baby rides. Many carriers include handy nursing flaps. These carriers are also great for fathers, who often enjoy carrying the baby around this way (and babies love being held against Daddy's big, warm chest).

stimulation of the outside world. You may be able to put him to sleep under a big shirt—very handy in restaurants, movie theaters, art museums, or anywhere else that doesn't appreciate a screaming baby. (Surprisingly, many mothers nursing young infants do quite well in the backs of movie theaters. Nursing in combination with the dark theater often puts a baby right to sleep.)

Before you spend a lot of money, survey your maternity

clothes and all your prepregnancy clothes. Separate out all the things that will make nursing easy, and then see what you are missing. Even if you already have everything you need, it won't hurt to buy a few nice things that you can put aside for when you come home from the hospital. Consider it a reward for you, and a gift for your baby.

Also consider beginning to purchase clothes in natural fabrics only. You will feel better wrapped in 100 percent breathable cotton than in 100 percent acrylic. You'll also want to read labels before you buy because clothes will get messy faster than you can imagine (almost every time your baby has a meal!). Dry clean only? "That stain, you ask? Oh, that's breastmilk again," you confide to your trusted dry cleaner, who is now making a fortune on your new breastfeeding wardrobe. Forget it! Washable silks, cottons, and other natural fabrics are the best way to go.

CREATING YOUR PERFECT NURSING HAVEN

Realistically, you can nurse anywhere, especially anywhere in your own home. However, you will most likely find it satisfying beyond words to have a nursing haven, a tailor-made corner of the home just for you and your baby, furnished with all the creature comforts. In fact, you might love your nursing haven so much that you will want to have several of them around the house.

The first step in creating the perfect nursing haven is to make a list of all the things that will be important to you when nursing. This list will change as you go along, of course. You can't be expected to know *everything* you will want before you have even given birth. But you do know your own personality, so go ahead and begin a list to make a good start. To help adapt your nursing haven to yourself and your family, take the following quiz, then check to see what kind of nursing haven suits you best.

THE NURSING HAVEN QUIZ

1. Which of the following best describes your household environment?

    A. *Highly populated, loud, boisterous, friendly, and active.*
    B. *Quiet, secluded, cozy, a private refuge.*
    C. *High-tech, plugged-in, wired, on-line, tuned-in.*
    D. *Sophisticated, cultured, tasteful, and elegant.*
    E. *Who sees it? You're never there!*

2. When you imagine nursing, how do you picture you and your baby?

    A. *The loving center of a large, supportive network of family and friends who share in your experience and can sit comfortably with you to chat or drink coffee while you nurse.*
    B. *Cocooned in your own cloistered space, warm, private, and completely sheltered from the outside world.*
    C. *Conveniently comfortable with easy access to outside communication, able to answer the phone, check your e-mail, or watch the news without disturbing your baby.*
    D. *Ensconced like a queen on her throne, enjoying all the comforts you and your heir so richly deserve.*
    E. *You honestly can't even imagine what nursing is like.*

3. Your family and friends would describe you as:

    A. *An extrovert, talkative, friendly, open.*
    B. *An introvert, quiet, shy around strangers, private.*
    C. *A thoroughly modern woman, interested in all the conveniences of our technological society.*
    D. *Someone who loves to be pampered, served, and adored.*
    E. *The last time you saw your family, you were rushing off to work. Your friends are your work colleagues and you live for your job.*

4. Your favorite meal is:

   A. A big, family-style Italian dinner with spaghetti and meat-balls, garlic bread, a huge salad, and a delicious red wine or dark, sparkling cider.
   B. A warm, simple soup, crusty French bread, and a good cheese.
   C. A cheeseburger, fries, and a milkshake from the closest drive-thru, or a pizza delivered to your door.
   D. Caviar, pâté de foie gras, and champagne. What else is there?
   E. Take-out Chinese.

5. The outfit you like best is:

   A. Leggings and a big, comfy, oversized top.
   B. A comfortable, flowing, floral-print dress.
   C. Blue jeans and a cotton T-shirt.
   D. Anything silk.
   E. Your best tailored suit.

6. If you could go anywhere on vacation, you would go:

   A. To Disneyworld!
   B. To a cozy cabin in the Rocky Mountains or a ski chalet in Switzerland.
   C. To a fancy, service-oriented hotel with all the modern conveniences in New York or Los Angeles.
   D. On a first-class, ultraluxury cruise to the Caribbean.
   E. To an exciting, foreign city like London, Paris, Tokyo, or Milan.

7. You would most like to spend your day off:

   A. On a family picnic . . . and why not invite all your friends, too? The more, the merrier!
   B. Curled up in your favorite chair with a quilt and a great novel.
   C. Surfing the Internet and catching up on unanswered e-mail.

D. *Being served breakfast in bed, then lounging all day until dinner at the best restaurant in town.*
E. *What exactly is a day off, again?*

8. A great birthday present for you might be:

   A. *A big gift basket of festive party food to share.*
   B. *A promise of an entire weekend of family-free peace, quiet, and solitude.*
   C. *A laptop computer.*
   D. *Diamonds.*
   E. *A cellular phone.*

9. The vehicle you would most like to drive is:

   A. *A minivan.*
   B. *A Range Rover.*
   C. *A Porsche.*
   D. *A Rolls Royce.*
   E. *A Jaguar.*

10. You love to read:

    A. *Women's magazines and family magazines.*
    B. *Victorian novels and mysteries.*
    C. *Science/technology magazines and contemporary nonfiction.*
    D. *Romance novels and travel and leisure magazines.*
    E. *Industry publications and business magazines.*

Now, survey your answers, determine which letter or letters you picked most often, and read below for the type of nursing haven that will probably make you and your baby happiest.

If you chose mostly A's: You are people-oriented and you like to be in the center of things. You might want to consider locating your nursing haven in a corner of the living room or family room where the baby can nurse while still being involved in whatever the family is doing. Include a comfortable chair with an ottoman or some type of footrest, a soft quilt, blanket, or shawl for warmth (and any necessary cover-up in the presence of company), a table to hold a beverage and a snack, and at least one other chair nearby for a friend or family member to pull close to yours, with access to a surface for refreshments. You might consider locating a second nursing haven in a more private location, such as your bedroom or the nursery, for those times when you want to escape the fray. Even for you, company can sometimes become overwhelming, especially in the first few weeks after you bring your baby home. And newborns are easily overstimulated by too much activity in the first few months, which can interfere with nursing.

If you chose mostly B's: You are a private person who enjoys quiet comfort away from the mainstream of activity. You love your friends and family, of course, but your soul requires occasional solitude to stay peaceful. Locate your nursing haven in a room where you can close the door and be alone, such as the nursery, the bedroom, or a study or guest room. Make sure to have a big, comfortable chair with a footrest, a quilt or blanket in a fabric you love, a table to hold a warm beverage (not hot, for your baby's safety), and a shelf to hold a selection of your favorite books. Make or buy a "Please Do Not Disturb" sign, as elaborate as you like, to hang on the door while you are nursing, so family members know to allow you this time alone. If you have a private deck or porch, you might want to consider setting up an alternate nursing haven outside (providing the weather is mild). Nursing in nature is relaxing and revitalizing. If you and your baby can enjoy peaceful seclusion in your nursing sessions together, you will both be better able to face the hectic pace of daily life.

If you chose mostly C's: You love the modern conveniences of life and you not only know how to program your VCR, but you are probably computer literate and your house is filled with the latest technology, including a home office. Locate your nursing

FATHER ALERT!

YOU ARE WELCOME TOO!

You can contribute to the magical atmosphere of your partner or spouse's nursing haven by volunteering to preserve and maintain it for as long as the haven is needed. Fluff cushions, alternate blankets, make custom cassettes for a portable tape player with music your partner and baby will love to nurse by. Leave loving and encouraging notes for her on the table by the nursing chair. Place a snack and a beverage on the table, waiting for your grateful partner to enjoy during a late-night feeding. (You might even want to install one of those mini refrigerators near the nursing haven and stock it with fruit and juices.)

Don't assume she will always want to be alone when nursing the baby. The nursing haven can be a haven for you, too. Sit with her and talk about your hopes, plans, and dreams. Brush her hair, feed her grapes, sing lullabyes together. How romantic!

haven near your desk where you have a phone and your computer. Choose a comfortable chair with armrests and wheels so you can scoot over to your desk, answer the phone, log in, receive and read a fax, and nurse all at once. Of course, sometimes you will want to relax and focus on your baby, but especially after you have been nursing for a while, and especially if you work at home, he won't mind if you get some things done, as long as he is with you and able to nurse. You will find a sling or infant carrier invaluable because it will keep your hands free. Don't forget a coaster on your desk to hold something to drink. You will probably want an alternative nursing haven away from your home office, too. Focusing on your baby and relaxing won't be easy at your desk. Set up a comfortable chair in the nursery or bedroom, and get away from it all at least once or twice a day.

If you chose mostly D's: You love luxury, and if you've been feeling good, you've loved being pregnant because of all the attention and help you get from everyone. Once you have your baby and much of the attention is shifted away from you and onto her, don't feel guilty about pampering yourself. Your nursing haven should be in your favorite room, in a luxuriously soft chair with an ottoman or, even better, a beautiful chaise. Always keep a soft blanket on the back of the chair (washable silk is wonderful), include a table to hold something to drink and a plate of your favorite healthy snack (imported cheese on crackers, cashew nuts, olives, strawberries dipped in real whipped cream), and be sure to keep lots of small pillows nearby for propping your head, arms, legs, feet, and baby, of course. Locate the nursing haven in a place where you won't be bothered by activity, noise, or family members asking for things. A source for music such as a stereo or portable cassette or CD player can add to the luxurious atmosphere, and your baby will surely benefit, too, if she nurses at the breast of a happy mother while listening to Mozart.

If you chose mostly E's: You immerse yourself in your work and are constantly busy. You love the fast pace and exciting rhythm of the working world, and may find it difficult to slow down and relax. Motherhood may come as a bit of a shock, but once you accustom yourself to your new role, you may find it is more rewarding than you could have imagined. Your nursing haven should be completely void of signs of work. Give yourself and your baby a break, and take advantage of your time together. Chances are you will be returning to work soon, so make the most of nursing. Choose a room that is quiet, with soft lighting and comfortable furnishings. Put your feet up. Focus on and touch your child. Wrap yourself in a blanket, savor a cup of

ELEMENTS OF A
PERFECT NURSING HAVEN

⊚ A comfortable chair that allows you to lean back and close your eyes.

⊚ An ottoman, footstool, or other soft surface on which to elevate your feet.

⊚ A quilt, comforter, blanket, or other soft covering in which to wrap yourself and your baby when it is cold, or just for the sense of security.

⊚ Lots of pillows in different sizes for propping your arms so you can effortlessly hold the baby to your breast, for supporting your head or neck, for relieving a strained lower back, or for propping under your knees and feet.

⊚ A small table or other accessible surface with a coaster for holding a beverage and a small plate for snacks. Getting yourself something to drink before you retire to your nursing haven is a good habit. Busy moms often forget to drink enough fluid, and adequate fluid intake is helpful to breastfeeding. Just be careful not to drink anything hot while holding your baby, for safety's sake.

⊚ A shelf to hold your favorite books, magazines, crossword puzzles, or other amusements.

⊚ A source of music and a few of your favorite CDs or tapes. Music can be relaxing for you and your baby, and a relaxed nursing couple is an effective nursing couple.

> ⊚ You and your baby. Your baby is utterly focused on you
> when nursing. Return the favor! You will always trea-
> sure this time, so make the most of every nursing
> moment.
>
> (Something to look back on when you have a difficult
> teenager on your hands!)

warm green tea, and bond with your baby. This is your chance to
begin a ritual that can start and end your work days in the future,
allowing your baby to say good-bye and then to greet you again
in an intimate and familiar way. These nursing sessions will
become an invaluable way for the two of you to keep in touch
once you return to work. Your nursing haven should facilitate
this goal by eliminating all mundane distractions.

Remember, your baby will sense if you aren't comfortable, so
make sure you tailor your nursing haven to be a place you
absolutely love.

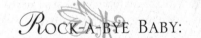 Rock-a-bye Baby: Where Your Baby Will Sleep

The question of where the baby will sleep is an important one for
a new family, and has some direct impact on the breastfeeding
relationship. Sleeping arrangements need to be manageable and
comfortable for everyone—mother, father, and little one. You may
find that once your baby arrives, all of your preconceived notions
about who sleeps where, why, and how, will fly out the window
as you all adapt to her personality and to your own impulses and
preferences. It's not too early, however, to start thinking about it.

There are as many variations on the whole sleep experience as there are new babies to love and nurture. We'll give you a selection of alternatives, incorporating, to a greater or lesser extent, the concept of the family bed. The family bed can be a viable (and practical!) suggestion for breastfeeding households. We know it may not be for everyone, and a family bed is certainly not required to ensure breastfeeding success, but you may find some variation useful and worth trying, if even for just those first few weeks or months. Keep an open mind and read on.

For some reason, our culture hasn't fully embraced the concept of the family bed. Indeed, the practice of having a baby sleep in a separate room is only about as old as the United States of America, and is widespread only in Western, industrialized nations. A family bed is simple. Mother, father, and baby sleep together. The baby can nurse to her heart's content and Mom can sleep right through it! When the baby wakes up, she is safely nestled between the two people she trusts. Waking up in the morning is lots of fun. You can nurse, and when the baby is full, she can turn to Dad for tickles and play. Mornings become a joyful and loving time for everyone in the family.

But won't the baby fall out of the bed? Might one of you roll over onto him? Will he ever learn to sleep alone? First of all, he won't be able to roll on his own for some time. (Babies can roll over, usually only one way, as early as two months old, but some don't accomplish this feat until as late as five months.) When he *can* roll over, however, a simple solution is to put him between you and a wall, or between you and your partner. Parents remain aware of their infants even when sleeping—it's a built-in instinct. You won't roll over on your baby. (However, *never* sleep with your infant or small child if you or your partner have been drinking alcohol or taking drugs—prescription or otherwise—that may impair your awareness.)

And no, the baby won't sleep with you forever. Anywhere from six months to the second or third year, your child will probably express a desire for his own crib or bed. If he is over thirty-six inches tall when he is ready for his own sleeping space, he may graduate straight to a bed because he is tall enough to climb out of a crib at this height (some vigorous climbers can accomplish this feat even earlier, so be aware of your child's tendencies).

Also, babies already at risk for sudden infant death syndrome (SIDS) may be better protected when sleeping with their parents. Earlier studies professing that infants sharing their parents' beds may have higher rates of SIDS have since been questioned, and more recent research refutes this claim, demonstrating that the opposite is more likely to be true. (However, SIDS *does* seem to occur more often in babies sleeping with parents who smoke.) Close proximity to the mother's sleep movements and sounds may cause a baby to wake up more often, which might help him to breathe more regularly, according to research being conducted at the University of California, Irvine, School of Medicine. This research suggests that mother's and baby's sleep patterns are meant to be intricately intertwined and mutually influenced. A baby left to his own devices may not sleep as well precisely because he wakes less often.

One caveat: The incidence of SIDs has decreased significantly since the medical community has made an effort to inform parents that babies should be put to sleep on their backs. Especially in the family bed, where softer mattresses and bedding may hinder breathing, putting baby to sleep on her back is particularly important.

You can certainly modify the family bed concept to fit your own family. Some mothers nurse their babies to sleep in the master bed, then move the sleeping infant to a bassinet or crib next to the bed, or to one that is placed in the corner of the parents' bedroom. Some families sleep together on a mattress or futon on the floor of the nursery until the baby is ready for the crib. Sometimes the baby will sleep in her own room and her parents will bring her into bed with them in the mornings when she wakes up, before the parents are ready to face the day. Other families invite

FATHER ALERT!

THERE'S A BABY IN THE BED!

The family bed, or some modification of it, can be a great opportunity for you to be intimately involved in the nursing process. Skin-to-skin contact is important to a baby. With Mom nursing and you holding your baby's hand, rubbing his back, or resting your hand on his head while holding Mom's hand, too, the entire family can share in the intimate experience of touch. Not only will your baby feel secure and loved by both of you, but Mom will really appreciate the contact and your support and involvement. In fact, a show of support like this will probably get you a really great back rub after the baby falls asleep! (Refer to the section on massage in chapter 7.)

the kids to sleep in the big bed only occasionally. Whatever works for your family is what you should practice. Your baby can have her own room all along, for changing, napping, and playing, which will make the move from family bed or a crib in the master bedroom to her own room—presented with all due fanfare and ceremony—much easier.

On the other hand, some families just aren't suited for the family bed, and some babies aren't, either. Nighttime feedings may be more comforting when they are performed in your nursing haven, and very small infants are more easily nursed when Mom is sitting upright anyway. Having a baby in the bed may distract you or your partner from getting any sleep at all, and the baby may sleep more restlessly, especially after the first few months. If she tosses and turns, then falls right to sleep when you move her to her crib, she is ready to sleep alone. If you go to sleep much later than the baby, you may not have anywhere to put her, especially once she is old enough to roll off the edge of the bed. Your baby may love having her own room and her own crib filled with his favorite toys and blankets. She will probably want you as soon as she wakes up (or she may like to play alone for a while), but she may want her own space in which to sleep. A baby monitor next to your bed (the monitor picks up every little noise) will put your mind at ease. Once again, get to know your baby! You should be able to sense what she wants. Be flexible. Arrangements can change nightly if it suits your family—or, your baby may not care where she sleeps as long as the place is consistent.

If you decide to have a family bed, will you and your partner still have a chance to be intimate? Of course. Be creative! You won't want to make love in the family bed when the baby is present—the family bed is for family—but there are a lot of other relatively comfy surfaces in the house besides the bed that can accommodate more couple-oriented activities. Try the couch, a blanket on the living room floor, a pile of pillows by a roaring fire, the shower or bathtub, or even a sleeping bag in the backyard under the stars! (Bring the baby monitor, just in case.) Who knows . . . the family bed could be just the revitalization your romantic life needs! See chapter 8 for a more detailed discussion of the effects of the breastfeeding life on your love life.

The Natural Home

Once you have a baby, you see the world differently. You may experience an increasing desire to make your home environment pure, clean, and natural. Consider the materials in your home. Consider your own clothing, your furniture, your carpets and rugs, curtains, floors, and wall coverings. Many of these things may be permanently fixed or too expensive to alter, but, if you can, think about replacing polyester with cotton, linen, and silk; plastic with wood; carpeting with hardwood flooring; and vinyl with ceramic where possible (and where practical). In addition, many natural materials are more durable and will last longer, so they are a better investment (e.g., high-quality wood furniture and ceramic tiles versus anything of particle board, plastic, or vinyl), and you will cut down on the incidence of airborne toxins in your home. New carpeting is a source of chemical toxins—if you've installed carpeting in the last six months, try to keep your house aired out as much as possible.

Another way to keep your house in harmony with nature is to fill it with living things. Plants, fish tanks, vases of fresh flowers, and other natural decorations add serenity to any living environment. Houseplants help to remove airborne toxins and fill your home with oxygen—and relaxing in front of a fish tank lowers blood pressure and reduces stress. Of course, don't take on any living creatures or elaborate plants you won't have time to maintain properly. Fish tanks must be cleaned and plants must be watered. Also, keep houseplants out of reach of toddlers, who are notorious for throwing, playing in, and eating dirt, just because it's there!

Especially make sure your baby's clothing, bedding, receiving blankets, linens, and toys are made primarily from natural fabrics. Or course, you have to be practical and consider what is washable, unbreakable, and easy to clean. Wooden rattles, washable silk blankets (easy to make), and natural cotton clothing will make her feel comfortable and you feel good. Let in natural light and fresh air whenever you can. Miniature, desk-top-sized fountains add moisture and the relaxing sounds of water to your home.

We probably don't even need to mention here (but we will, anyway!) that a household with smokers is a household with polluted air. Babies whose parents smoke have far higher rates of asthma and other respiratory problems, and may have an increased chance of dying from sudden infant death syndrome (SIDS). Smoking and babies don't mix. Ask your doctor about the best ways to quit smoking.

HOME IS WHERE YOUR HEART IS

Bringing your new baby home is a special moment in the life of your family—perhaps the most important one since you and your partner or spouse decided to set out on a life together. Use this time before your new addition arrives to work together as a team to create the kind of home atmosphere you've always dreamed of for yourselves and your child, one that will accommodate your family's breastfeeding and living style. What better way to express your love for each other, and for your new baby, than to create a thoughtfully functional, warm, and supportive environment for the whole family?

3

Breastfeeding Basics
for New Mothers

Getting to Know Your Baby

*A*FTER the long months of preparation and the frantic rush of labor and delivery, many parents don't think about the actuality of bringing home a brand new person who will live with them and depend on them for the next twenty years or so—a person they don't even know! Every baby is different and the first few weeks of having the new baby at home will be weeks of great celebration and of great transition. You will be surprised by your new baby on a daily basis.

The arrangement may seem temporary to you, or even unreal. How could this tiny person belong to you? How could you have made him? What will she be like? What is he thinking? What does she want? Your baby's needs are simple: you. A new baby needs to have his mother close to him, nursing him, touching him, kissing him, attending to his needs. A new baby also wants her father to hold her, talk to her, play with her, bathe her, rock her to sleep. Your baby, however, will not be the same as your sister's baby or the baby down the street, or even the same as you were when you were a baby (according to the stories this little one will surely inspire in the new grandparents). You all need time to

FATHER ALERT!

GREAT WAYS TO WELCOME HOME A NEW MOTHER

You've both been through a lot, and you may feel neglected in the rush, or you may still be reeling, or you may be utterly smitten with your new child. Remember, however, that suddenly, all the attention that has been lavished on your partner for the past nine months has now been transferred to the baby. A new mother may be feeling euphoric, but this may dip unexpectedly into the blues faster than you can say "post-partum depression." If you make a fuss about welcoming your partner home, you will make her happy. Customize the fuss to her personality, but don't think she doesn't want it. She'll be touched. Here are some ideas:

- Bring her a big bouquet of seasonal flowers, or a single white rose, which symbolizes purity and is evocative of the new little one.

- Arrange for a friend to have dinner prepared and the table set with your good china and candles. Serve her.

- Buy something for the baby, and have it gift-wrapped. If you aren't sure what to get a baby, it probably doesn't matter—your partner will be touched that you made the gesture—but anything from a simple baby rattle to a fancy musical mobile is appropriate.

- Buy your partner something engraved with the baby's name, initials, or the names of all the family members.

- Jewelry with the baby's birthstone, perhaps together with hers and yours—the new family!—is always welcome.

⦿ The first night home, after the baby falls asleep, brush your partner's hair and give her a foot rub. Tell her you are proud of her. (But hurry—new babies don't stay asleep for long!)

adjust to each other and learn about each other. Your baby may sleep endlessly, or hardly at all. She may want to nurse every hour, or she may need to be coaxed to nurse because she is too busy examining her new world. He may love to be cuddled while nursing, or he may be a squirmer. Whatever your baby's personality, don't expect her to fit into your preconceived notions of how a baby should act, or to adapt to your rigidly prearranged breastfeeding schedule. Your baby is a person in her own right! Take the time to get to know her.

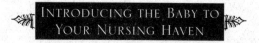

INTRODUCING THE BABY TO YOUR NURSING HAVEN

When you first bring your baby into his new home, you'll want to give him a tour and introduce him, carefully, to his new siblings and family pets. The stimulation of the trip home from the hospital and arriving in a new place will be a lot for your newborn to absorb, so be gentle and take your time. Once the baby has seen his new environment, head directly to your nursing haven for some much-needed comforting, feeding, and revitalizing for both you and your baby. If your infant has an older brother or sister, he or she can spend this time with Dad preparing a special surprise for Mom and the baby to celebrate the first nursing session at home, such as making a "welcome to the family" card for the baby or preparing a delicious blended fruit smoothie for Mom to enjoy and help her stay hydrated while feeding the new baby.

PETS ARE FAMILY TOO

Family pets experience a big transition when a new baby arrives. To help ready your pet, bring home a receiving blanket that the baby has been wrapped in (don't wash it) and let your pet sniff it, even sleep with it, a day or two before the baby comes home. Then, the new baby won't smell so strange and unfamiliar.

Some mothers take to breastfeeding right away. Probably more often, however, mothers who are new to breastfeeding are a little nervous when they first bring home that tiny, delicate creature. Your breastfeeding "comfort level" is partly a function of your personality. Also, mothers who have read up on the subject, taken a prenatal baby-care class, or joined a support group tend to feel a little more comfortable. If you feel jittery about doing everything correctly, even if you *have* read all the books and attended the classes, try to relax. Listen to your instincts and do what feels right. Also, keep a few good books about child care handy for quick reference (this book, plus see Appendix B, "Resources," which begins on page 271) and post your pediatrician's number near every phone. Don't ever be afraid to call your pediatrician to ask a question about breastfeeding or baby care.

We've mentioned before how prolactin in your system will enhance your maternal feelings, just one more advantage of breastfeeding. Maternal feelings aren't everything, though. Practice counts for a lot, so rest assured that, although you may feel unsure and tentative on how to go about breastfeeding right now, in a few weeks you'll be a pro. Ask questions of all your visiting friends and relatives who are mothers. Above all, touch and hold and nurse your newborn as often as possible. He'll let you know what he needs.

CESAREAN SECTIONS CAN BE BREASTFEEDING-FRIENDLY

Women who have had a cesarean section can still breastfeed. If you are scheduled to have a cesarean section, or if your obstetrician decides during delivery that a cesarean section is advisable, be sure to alert the physician and the anesthesiologist that you will be breastfeeding. They will choose drugs for the procedure that will allow you to begin breastfeeding as soon as you are physically able, awake, and alert after surgery. Be comforted to know that the American Academy of Pediatrics asserts that the benefits to a baby of breastfeeding outweigh the risks of his drowsiness from the effect of post-surgery analgesics—or pain relievers (even narcotics)—your physician prescribes for you. Be sure to let your physician know that you want to have time with your baby immediately after giving birth. You'll want to hold your baby in breast-feeding positions that are comfortable for your postsurgery body such as the football hold (see step 3, on the next page). Breastfeeding soon after delivery will even aid in your healing by helping your uterus to contract more quickly.

THE BREASTFEEDING TECHNIQUE

While you were still in the hospital, immediately after delivery, your breasts felt soft at first but quickly began to engorge and become full. The more you nursed your infant, starting in the hospital or birthing center soon after delivery, the fuller your breasts became. In the first four or five days postpartum, your breast produce the nutrient-rich colostrum, for feeding.

During the first week after giving birth, the body starts to mix the colostrum with an increasing amount of mature breast-milk until the breastmilk completely replaces it. By now you may be home with the baby and you will notice the difference as the colostrum gives way to the production of breastmilk—a process known as having your milk "come in."

So, How Do You Do It?

Following these twelve steps will make for an easy breastfeeding beginning for you and your baby.

1. *Get something to drink.* A glass of water, juice, low-fat milk, or soy milk will help hydrate you and facilitate breastmilk production.

2. *Make yourself and your baby comfortable.* Settle into your nursing haven or other comfortable location. Place the baby in position for nursing. In every position, remember that he should be able to feed without having to turn his head; face his entire body towards you. His mouth should move straight towards your breast. Rotating positions with each nursing will help to drain the milk ducts more evenly.

3. *Relax.* Take a few deep breaths, close your eyes, and concentrate on becoming calm and quiet. Imagine all your stress melting away.

Here are three positions to try:

The Cradle Hold.
⊚ *Sit well supported so you aren't hunkered over the baby; place a pillow under the baby for cushioning and rest your feet on a footstool, coffee table, or any elevated surface (even a pile of child care books!), to bring her up against your breast without having to lean your body forward. Her tiny body will be perpendicular and face-*

to-face with yours, with one of her arms under your breast and one over. Support her with her head in the crook of your elbow and her hips resting in your hand.

The "Nurse-N-Doze."

◎ *Lie down on your side with your baby beside you. If you need extra support, you can place some pillows between your knees, behind you, or under your head and shoulders. While he faces you, cradle his head with your free arm; your bottom arm should be folded up under your head, comfortably out of the way. If the baby needs help to reach your nipple straight on, place a small pillow or a folded baby blanket under his head so you don't have to reach your breast down and he doesn't have to reach his mouth up. This is a great position for late night and early morning feedings—or any time you feel like resting completely, and easiest with larger babies. It's also a good position for mothers who have had cesarean section deliveries—especially while still in the hospital and recovering from surgery.*

The Football Hold.

◎ *Put a pillow next to you. Rest the baby on her back on the pillow. Cradle her head with your hand and her body on your forearm so her feet point behind you, toward your elbow. Bring the baby close, holding her against your side. The football hold is a good position for mothers who've had cesarean sections because it places no pressure on the abdomen; it's also good for breastfeeding multiples and premature or smaller infants (See pages 62–67).*

4. *Brush your nipple against your's baby's cheek.* This stimulates the rooting reflex, a baby's instinctual response to find a nipple. Once he is comfortable with nursing, you won't need to signal in this way, but at first he needs your guidance. He's

never done this, either! If you are waking him from sleep for a feeding, you might want to try expressing a few drops of milk onto his mouth to whet his appetite. Also try brushing your nipple up and down over his lips.

5. *Draw the baby close to you* as she opens her mouth to find your breast. Gently holding your areola, direct it towards the center of her mouth while you pull her closer, so she can latch on to the entire areola and not just the nipple. Bring the baby close to the breast, not the breast close to the baby. As soon as she opens wide, place her firmly on the breast.

   If your baby latches onto the wrong place or doesn't get enough of the nipple, insert your finger into the corner of her mouth to break the suction and pull her gently away. Try again until she has a good, firm hold and little, if any, of the areola is showing.

6. *Make sure the baby can breathe.* Newborns are small and your engorged breast can sometimes block a baby's nose. Whenever this happens, either lean back a bit to give him breathing room, or gently place your finger between his nose and you to make some space.

7. *Watch for a rhythmic sucking motion.* Breastfeeding is laborious work for a brand new baby, though well worth the effort. She should look like she is sucking hard. After you feel the milk ejection reflex, when letdown begins, you should be able to hear her gulping and swallowing. If your milk comes out so fast that she begins to choke, break the suction, express a little milk, and start again. (Don't be surprised if your breasts "spout" when you first take the baby off.) Also, it is common for a baby to spit up breastmilk while nursing, particularly if she is gulping aggressively. It's O.K. Forceful vomiting, however, is another matter and should be reported to your pediatrician.

8. *Alternate the starting breast with every feeding.* This prevents one breast from becoming painfully engorged, and assures a well-established milk supply in both breasts. If you don't remember every time, that's all right, and even if you aren't sure, you may be able to feel which breast is fuller. Switching a watch, ring, bracelet, or even a piece of ribbon around your wrist or bra strap after each nursing to remind you where to start works for many mothers. If your baby shows a preference for feeding at one breast more than the other, try rotating nursing positions with each feeding as well, to help keep your little one from insisting on a one-sided routine.

9. *Support your breast with your hand (the one that isn't holding the baby!) in a comfortable fashion if it won't stay in place.* While you are in a seated position to feed your baby, you'll want to hold your breast in a comfortable position. You can keep your hand in the same grasp you used to bring him to your breast, with the four fingers of your hand supporting your breast and your thumb above the areola. Or you can use the scissors grasp, in which three fingers remain under the breast for support and the thumb and forefinger are placed over the areola. Use whichever grasp feels best to you, but remember to keep your fingers away from the areola; he needs to be able to take it fully into his mouth and he can't if your fingers are in the way.

10. *Work up to about ten or fifteen minutes on the first breast* at each feeding. Before your milk comes in, five minutes is sufficient, but after that point, ten minutes on the first breast, then allowing the baby to nurse as long as desired on the other side, will assure that each breast is mostly emptied and this, too, will help to establish a plentiful milk supply. If your baby falls asleep too quickly, try holding her upright, lightly tapping the bottom of her foot, or talking to her while you nurse. If she snoozes despite your efforts, nurse more often

Is Your Baby Getting Enough Milk?

If your baby is gaining weight and seems healthy, chances are good that plenty of nourishment is being received. Just in case, however (because you'll worry about it no matter what), here are some things to look for, all signs that a baby is adequately nourished. If you have any doubt at all, don't be afraid to call your pediatrician.

◎ The baby wets eight to ten diapers in a twenty-four-hour period, and the urine is light in color (dark urine signals dehydration). The ultra-absorbent disposables are hard to gauge, but check for heaviness every couple of hours, or take a peek inside and look for discoloration.

◎ The baby has at least five and up to twelve bowel movements in a twenty-four-hour period. About four days after birth the stool will appear yellow, loose, and seedy; this is the normal appearance of breastfed stool. Before this, however, right after birth, a dark green-black substance called meconium is passed, which is followed about the third day by a green-brown stool. (Babies vary greatly in their bowel habits. If you are worried, call your pediatrician.)

◎ When you nurse, you feel the tingling sensation of the milk ejection reflex (sometimes it takes a few minutes), after which your baby gulps and swallows vigorously, a sign that her sucking is properly triggering your breasts to produce adequate milk (see page 10–11 for a more detailed discussion of the process of milk production). Also, when your milk first came in, your breasts became engorged.

⊚ The baby nurses for at least ten minutes on one breast, then five to ten minutes on the other breast, every two to three hours for the first few weeks. Thereafter, she nurses on demand. (Longer stretches during the night or occasional days when your baby wants to nurse more often are both normal.)

⊚ The baby latches on well and after the first few weeks, nursing is completely painless and feels "right."

If your baby just isn't gaining weight, call your pediatrician. It is normal for your baby to lose weight immediately after birth. However, within ten days, the infant should be back to her birth weight and consistently gaining thereafter, at a rate of about an ounce per day for the first couple of months. Problems in gaining weight are commonly remedied by trying a new feeding position, or by revising the feeding schedule or the frequency of feedings. Your physician will closely monitor the situation until your baby is back on track and gaining weight at an acceptable pace.

to maintain your milk supply and keep her gaining weight. But don't worry if every feeding isn't exactly ten minutes—it's just a guideline.

11. *Bond with your baby and, whenever it seems right, involve the family.* Once your baby is nursing comfortably, enjoy your time together. Talk to her, look at her, examine her tiny hands and feet. Cuddle together. This is the way mother and baby become intimately acquainted. That little stranger will become part of you in no time. The newborn stage is so short, you'll want to savor it.

If Dad is nearby, invite him to cuddle with you. And if older children are curious, bring them into your circle, too.

This is a good time to share stories with your baby's siblings about their own births, feeding histories, and infancy experiences. Kids love to hear stories about themselves, and are fascinated to learn about things they can't remember.

Sometimes you will want to nurse in privacy, but a big family cuddle can be renewing, and will help to foster positive attitudes about breastfeeding in every family member. Keeping this in mind, you also won't want to force anyone to participate who isn't willing. Respect each person's space and adjustment period.

12. *Don't put them away wet (your breasts, that is) and remember to burp the baby.* After you nurse, dry your nipples before returning them to their dark and poorly ventilated home inside your bra. If you have the privacy, pat them dry and give them some air (i.e., leave them exposed for a while), which will help to toughen the skin and minimize nipple soreness.

    Breastfed babies generally swallow less air than ones who are bottle-fed, so burping may not be quite as elaborate a ritual for breastfeeding couples! However, she should be burped after finishing at one breast and before being offered the other. To burp, hold your baby upright against your chest with her head above your shoulder and pat her *gently on the back*. Make sure to put a towel or cloth over your shoulder to catch any spit-up (this practice will quickly become a reflex action).

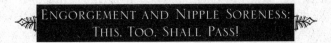

ENGORGEMENT AND NIPPLE SORENESS:
THIS, TOO, SHALL PASS!

The first few weeks of breastfeeding can be physically trying. Your breasts are so swollen and hard, they feel like they weigh ten pounds each. Your nipples may be cracked and sore, and when your baby latches on, it may feel like a sandpaper rub. Your

EXPRESSING BREASTMILK MANUALLY

Learning how to express breastmilk from your breasts using just your own hands is well worth the effort. As in breastfeeding itself, you'll need to take a little time and practice a lot. A lactation consultant can help you perfect your technique. If you have a friend who is also breastfeeding her baby and knows how to express milk manually, and you both feel comfortable about it, ask her to show you how she does it—a picture is worth a thousand words. For now, though, here in plain English is how to go about it:

◉ Wash your hands carefully with disinfectant soap. Use a nailbrush to scrub under your fingernails.

◉ Clean and sterilize (boil for five minutes) a cup, bowl, or baby bottle (you'll want to sterilize a wide-mouth funnel as well if you are expressing into a baby bottle). Hold it under your breast to collect the breastmilk.

◉ Place the fingers of your free hand around your areola as if you are beginning to nurse your baby. The thumb is over the top of the areola and the finger underneath. For expressing milk, you'll want your fingers to be about an inch or two behind the nipple.

◉ Using the thumb and the first two fingers under your breast, push the breast back against your chest. Avoid cupping your breast in your hand or squeezing the breast too vigorously, which could hurt and may cause bruises.

◉ Stroke your breast on all sides towards the nipple to encourage milk movement, alternately pressing with your thumb and fingers at the base of the areola in a repeated rhythm to begin expressing milk. Move your hand clockwise, then counterclockwise, around the breast to empty as many milk ducts as possible. Alternating hands to express the breastmilk is another way to make sure you are emptying milk evenly from the breast.

◎ Express milk for a few minutes—three to five is perfect—from each breast and then repeat. You should be able to express an ounce or two of milk manually, using this method.

Expressed breastmilk fed to a baby within thirty minutes requires no special storage. If you will use the milk within 24 hours, you can place it in *sterile,* four-ounce plastic nursing bottles and refrigerate or store in a cooler. Whatever the baby does not consume during a feeding should be thrown away. Don't reuse expressed milk or leave it sitting around. Using a breast pump is the fastest, most efficient way to express breastmilk. For more on pumping and storing breastmilk, see page 88.

baby may have trouble latching on when your breast is engorged. Your breasts are adjusting, just like the rest of you, while your baby is learning the ropes. Be assured that this discomfort will soon pass, and you will be nursing effortlessly and with great pleasure very soon. In the meantime, here are a few suggestions:

◎ *Wear your bra, even to bed. At first, engorgement makes any breast movement painful. Keeping your breasts secure in a good nursing bra minimizes movement.*

◎ *To ease engorgement, manually express or pump some of your milk before your baby feeds. (See "Expressing Breastmilk Manually" above or "Breast Pump Choices" on page 91.) This can help a lot if* you are uncomfortable but your baby isn't awake or ready to eat yet (common in the morning if he slept through the night without nursing), or if you are so engorged that your baby is having difficulty latching on. Don't worry about using up your milk. The more you use, the more you'll make.

◎ A warm shower, warm compresses, ice packs, expressing milk, and gentle breast massage can all relieve engorgement pain. You might try a combination.

◎ Make a concerted effort to nurse every two to three hours as recommended for the first six weeks. It's the best plan for your newborn and for your breasts. If you go for longer periods between feedings, engorgement will recur, your milk production may drop off, and your baby make take longer to gain weight.

◎ To make nursing more comfortable and more profitable for the baby, make sure she latches on correctly. In essence, she needs to open wide and take the entire nipple and areola into her mouth. If she is just sucking on the nipple, it will hurt! (And she won't get enough milk, either.) Avoid pushing her face into your breast or pressing on her cheeks as tactics to get her to latch on; they won't work and will only upset her. Your goal is to get your baby to open wide, then bring her firmly to the breast so she can latch on correctly. Focus on accessing her rooting reflex (see step 4 on page 50), which causes her to want to suck and draw in the nipple and areola. Tickle her lips or cheek with your nipple after expressing a little milk, to give her a taste of what's coming and encourage her cooperation.

◎ Avoid using devices such as nipple shields, which interfere with a baby's correct stimulation of the nipple.

◎ Just as when you were pregnant, don't wash your nipples with soap or apply any lotions or creams. Instead, express a little milk *and rub it into your nipples. Soap will dry and irritate the skin, exacerbating any soreness you may have. Expose your breasts to the air whenever possible, and wash them with water only. (Remember, the Montgomery glands will take care of germs, so you don't need soap.) And once again, if your nipple are very dry, you can rub in a little vegetable oil.*

◎ *Remember to rotate nursing positions with each feeding. (See step 3 on page 49.) Evidence is mounting that the nursing position is a vital component to achieving nursing success for healthy breasts and a healthy baby. Don't let your baby continue to nurse if he isn't latched on correctly. Take him off the breast and try again. Cracked nipples, for example, are often a result of poor positioning.*

◎ *Even if you and your baby are doing everything right, you may still be a little sore for a while. Your nipples aren't used to this much activity! They will adjust, however, so bear with it; remember all the advantages colostrum and breastmilk are giving your baby (reread chapter 1 if you need to), and hold onto the fact (yes, fact!) that your nipples won't be sore for long.*

◎ *If you notice a small, painful red lump, possibly with red streaks radiating from it, you probably have a clogged milk duct. Nurse as much as possible on the affected breast (even if it hurts—emptying the duct promotes healing), and monitor yourself for symptoms of mastitis (see box on the next page). Warm compresses can be soothing.*

THE PLEASURES OF THE 2:00 A.M. FEEDING (REALLY!)

Pregnant women often dread the 2:00 A.M. feeding, and why shouldn't they? They've heard the stories of pacing the halls for hours with a colicky baby, they've seen the sleepless, haggard

WHEN TO CALL YOUR DOCTOR

◉ If you experience extreme pain, tenderness, redness, or burning; if your breast feels hard and swollen, even after nursing; or if you have aches, fever, and chills. These are all symptoms of mastitis, a breast infection that is painful and requires treatment. If you do get mastitis, it is important to keep nursing on the infected breast as frequently as possible, to ease the pressure and promote healing. In rare cases, untreated mastitis can lead to hospitalization. If you can possibly bring the baby with you to the hospital and continue nursing, do it. Otherwise, premature weaning may result. The infection will not affect your baby in any way. Your milk isn't infected.

◉ If you start to feel extremely depressed, have violent or self-destructive feelings, or don't feel any urge to feed or care for your baby. A few women experience serious postpartum depression, which is caused by hormones and is easily treated. Don't feel guilty about these feelings. You can't control your hormones, but medication can.

faces of new mothers and fathers, they know what a premium new parents place on opportunities to rest and revitalize. There is another side to the 2:00 A.M. feeding, however. Awake with your baby in the middle of the night, you can share a special time without distraction. You will always remember this very personal time with great pleasure and nostalgia. Here are some ways to enjoy these middle-of-the-night sessions:

◉ *Create a ritual. Keep a pitcher of water or juice in the refrigerator and pour yourself a tall glass before you fetch the baby (warm herbal tea or cocoa are cozy, but never drink a hot beverage while holding your baby). Wrap the two of you in a special quilt or blanket reserved just for 2:00 A.M. Keep a special book, tape, or CD on hand that you read or listen to only during this feeding. Softly read aloud or sing to the baby.*

◎ *Gaze into your baby's eyes. Sing lullabyes to him. Stroke his head. Tell him how much you love him. Revel in the euphoria of nursing.*

◎ *Find out what kind of weird programs are on TV at 2:00 A.M., and be amused by them (but keep the sound low, so the atmosphere stays peaceful and conducive to relaxation).*

◎ *Dream about what your infant will be like when she is two, six, twelve, fifteen, twenty years old.*

◎ *If weather and mosquitoes permit (or if you are lucky enough to have a screened-in porch), set up a nursing haven outside. Listen to the sounds of the night.*

◎ *Consider the family bed (see page 37), or some variation of it, which will allow you and your partner almost uninterrupted sleep while still satisfying the baby's needs for nourishment. Everyone will wonder why you look so rested!*

SPECIAL BREASTFEEDING CIRCUMSTANCES

There are some situations that make breastfeeding more of a challenge—but usually not impossible! Your determination to breastfeed your baby will give her all the benefits of breastmilk, as well as the support of the indescribable physical and emotional bond to you that nursing from your breast provides. Gather your health care team and your support group of family and friends close around you; they'll create a protective embrace of love and support for the breastfeeding team that will help carry you through. Remember why you wanted to begin breastfeeding in the first place, and hang in there. You'll be glad you did!

BREASTFEEDING YOUR PREMATURE BABY

A baby that is born before thirty-seven weeks' gestation is considered premature; today, approximately 10 percent of babies born in the United States are born prematurely. Depending upon your baby's size and condition, you may or may not be able to nurse her immediately from your own breast. However, you can surely give her the benefits of breastmilk by pumping milk that will be fed to her by you and/or hospital staff (see "Breast Pump Choices" in chapter 4). Many hospitals will make efficient electrical breast pumps available to you for free or for a small rental fee. Sometimes, premature babies can be fed from a "milk pool" created from the breastmilk of other new mothers who are pro-

BREASTMILK MAY BOOST A BABY'S BRAIN POWER

A British study of three hundred children born prematurely showed that the ones who were breastfed, or who received breastmilk supplemented by formula, scored higher on IQ tests than the ones who'd been bottle-fed. In addition, children whose mothers breastfed the longest had the highest IQs. Breastfed children averaged 103.7 points, while bottle-fed children averaged 93.1.

ducing more milk than their babies need. But this milk, intended for full-term babies, will not be as beneficial to her as *your* breastmilk will. Your milk has an enzyme called lipase that facilitates fat absorption in her tiny body—this process will help her to gain weight faster and reach the necessary five pounds she'll need to come home with her parents. The breastmilk of mothers who deliver prematurely also has more nitrogen, protein, lactose, sodium, and chloride. And don't forget about the wonderful advantages of colostrum!

Studies show that breastfeeding your premature baby ensures that she will receive the combination of nutrients most suited to her needs—your decision to breastfeed is one invaluable contribution you can make to your premature baby's health and well-being. Premature babies who are not fed with breastmilk are given high-protein formulas to help them grow faster. Researchers, however, have discovered that these formulas can be problematic because some babies' tiny bodies can't process the end products produced by the high-protein formula, causing potential health complications. Formulas are best used only as a supplement to your own breastmilk. Furthermore, the increased levels of prolactin in your bloodstream when you breastfeed are also passed along to your premature baby; new research shows that the breastfed baby's higher levels of prolactin contribute to decreased time on respirators and facilitate weight gain. Once again, your own breast is best!

If you begin breastfeeding your premature baby from birth, you'll be best able to continue to breastfeed at home. Remember, if you don't begin breastfeeding or pumping breastmilk soon after birth, you'll begin to lose the ability to produce breastmilk and it will be harder to stimulate the milk flow. If, for some reason, your physician advises against feeding her breastmilk for a short time, you can continue to pump and freeze your milk for future use.

When the time comes to begin breastfeeding your baby from your own breast, you'll want to be gentle and patient. He may not be able to latch on firmly or suck very hard at first. You may want to try expressing some milk initially to stimulate the milk ejection reflex, making it easier for him to receive the full flow of your milk, though chances are just looking at your baby or hearing him cry will do the trick.

If your baby doesn't seem interested in nursing, remember he's been through a lot and needs reassurance and encouragement. The closeness to your baby during these first attempts to nurse is as important as mastering the technique. You'll both get it—don't worry! At first, you can try positioning the baby so that you're holding him with the arm and hand opposite the breast you are feeding from. Support your breast with your free hand. The football hold is also good for small babies, and allows you eye-to-eye contact. (See page 50.)

Once you bring your baby home, you and your spouse or partner will want to give her lots of skin-to-skin contact and loving care. She's had the benefit of the best our state-of-the-art medical technology can provide, but nothing can substitute for the connection of touch and human contact, lovingly administered by her parents. Hold her, kiss her, keep her near you both. Remember that breastfeeding your premature baby is giving her many health advantages. Don't give up! Mothers of premature babies will tell you that the effort of keeping your milk in plentiful supply is well worth the effort as you watch your baby grow stronger and more robust with each passing day. Before they celebrate their first birthdays, most premature babies have already caught up with full-term babies.

MULTIPLES—A BREAST FOR EVERY BABY?

Surprise! You didn't just have a baby . . . you had two! (Or three? four? no, not . . . seven?!) Moms and Dads blessed with multiples will probably be overwhelmed with competing emotions. While they worry about finances, juggling schedules, and being able to accomplish even simple, basic baby care, they may also be elated, excited, and proud. After all, multiple births are relatively rare, and carrying and giving birth to multiple babies is an accomplishment extraordinaire.

But what about breastfeeding multiple babies? There are many compelling advantages to breastfeed both (or all!) your bundles of joy:

◉ *Many multiples are smaller than single babies, and often come ear- lier. Smaller and earlier babies can benefit even more dramatically from the nutrients, immunities, and other valuable substances in colostrum and breastmilk.*

◉ *Formula for two babies? You had better have a big savings account! Breastfeed, and spend your money on extra diapers or a diaper service.*

◉ *The more you breastfeed, the more milk you will produce. Mothers breastfeeding multiples don't have to worry about their milk sup- ply diminishing from lack of sufficient sucking. Twins will keep the milk flowing nicely, thank you. You'll want to make sure you get enough fluids to stay hydrated while breastfeeding—and you may find that you'll be hungrier, too! After all, you need to keep your own physical resources replenished as you nourish your babies, and you will need about 400-500 additional calories beyond the 500 extra you need to breastfeed one baby.*

◉ *Parents of multiples are often overwhelmed with the workload, and breastfeeding will force you to sit down and relax every few hours, a necessity for a new mother if she is to keep her health. You will need help, so hire someone, if your budget allows (or convince a rel- ative or friend), to help keep the house in order.*

◉ *You can nurse both babies at once (tandem nursing), or one after the other (make sure each gets to start on a full breast). The former method saves time and is fun but takes some practice and lots of pil- lows for propping; the latter method allows you to lavish all your attention on one baby at a time. You may want to try it both ways.*

If you do have multiples and are breastfeeding (or know you are carrying multiples and want to breastfeed), good for you! (And even better for your babies!) But find a support group. Multiple babies can reduce even the most organized and efficient parents to occasional tears. Look for groups of parents with multiples in your area, or start your own group. Or, call the La Leche League in your area. One of the best resources you can have is other parents in the same situation.

FATHER ALERT!

THE FAMILY LEAVE ACT

In February 1993, President Clinton signed the 1993 Family Leave Act, which requires employers with more than fifty employees to provide up to twelve weeks of unpaid leave to employees upon the birth or adoption of a child, or to care for ill family members. One of the benefits of this law is that you can take "paternity leave." Although many new fathers may not be able to take advantage of the law because they can't afford to miss that all-important paycheck (especially if Mom has taken unpaid leave or quit her job), those who can stay home for at least a week or two with their new babies shouldn't hesitate. Not only does your partner need the help, but you can participate more thoroughly and intensely in the early bonding process. Bathing, dressing, and playing with the baby, giving infant massages, cuddling with Mom during nursing, and taking your baby for walks are all great ways for you to be involved in your new child's life. Participate in baby care as much as possible. Being a full-time father for the first few weeks will help you get comfortable with your new family and with infant care.

BREASTFEEDING YOUR ADOPTED BABY

Believe it or not, you may be able to breastfeed your adopted baby. It takes some work, but it could be one of the most rewarding feats you will ever accomplish. If you are already nursing a toddler, stepping up your milk supply by additional breast pumping in preparation for the new baby's arrival is the easiest way to breastfeed an adopted baby. Even if you have never been pregnant, however, you can induce lactation in your breasts.

One of the problems with preparing to breastfeed an adopted baby is that many parents don't know exactly when they will bring their baby home. Sometimes, the call comes just a day or two before the happy event. However, if you do know when he will arrive, you can start using a breast pump or your hands to pump your breast for five minutes, three or four times every day (see "Expressing Breastmilk Manually" on page 56 or "Breast Pump Choices" on page 91). With some persistence, almost all breasts will eventually begin to produce milk.

A few women have nursed adopted babies without any formula supplementation, but others have found supplementation necessary. Even if your baby's diet is rounded out with formula, he will still be receiving wonderful benefits from your breastmilk, not to mention the emotional benefits of this close physical contact with you. An option for formula feeding is to use a device called a nursing supplementer. The supplementer holds bottles of formula (or pumped breastmilk). Thin tubes with valves on the ends are taped to the breasts, so the baby drinks from the tubes, which are against the nipple, while simultaneously nursing from the breast.

Although induced lactation can be difficult, perhaps the more imposing barrier is the attitude you may encounter about breastfeeding your adopted baby. A lot of people will think it is strange. We would like to offer the following: So what? As long as you and your immediate family are committed to the idea, know that what is best for your baby is far more important than what anyone else thinks.

For additional support, tell your doctor you are interested in induced lactation (it will help to find a doctor who is familiar with the idea and supports your decision), and talk to a lactation consultant and/or your local La Leche League for additional support and information. The La Leche League publishes a booklet about breastfeeding adopted children.

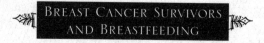

BREAST CANCER SURVIVORS AND BREASTFEEDING

If you are one of the small but growing number of women who experience breast cancer when still in their childbearing years, and you have had a mastectomy or lumpectomy combined with radiation therapy in one breast, you will still be able to breastfeed from the healthy breast. Research is inconclusive about whether breastfeeding is advantageous or disadvantageous to the breastfeeding mother, but generally it is thought to have some benefit. There is no evidence that breastfeeding passes on cancer, or conditions that foster a predisposition to cancer, to a baby through breastmilk. While most knowledge regarding premenopausal breast cancer survivors, pregnancy, and breastfeeding is still anecdotal, the prevailing opinion of researchers indicates that your long-term survival rate and your risk of recurrence of breast cancer do *not* increase by becoming pregnant or by breastfeeding.

It was once thought that a premenopausal breast cancer survivor should not become pregnant or breastfeed for three to five years after recovery because the hormones, most particularly estrogen, activated by pregnancy and breastfeeding might reactivate the cancer. This is now considered by most to be an unwarranted fear, but you will want to consult your physician and health care team to make the best decision for your particular medical circumstances.

Should you experience a recurrence of breast cancer while pregnant or breastfeeding, your physician will likely advise immediate surgery to remove the malignancy as a life-saving measure for you. Breastfeeding during adjuvant therapies—radiation or chemotherapy—is not advised. One of the first major studies examining the controversial issue of pregnancy, breastfeeding, and the premenopausal breast cancer survivor is being conducted by Memorial Sloan-Kettering Cancer Institute in New York City.

If you are a premenopausal woman who has survived breast cancer, is pregnant, and wants to breastfeed, make sure you have the full support of your health care team—including your obstetrician, pediatrician, breast cancer surgeon, and oncologist. Do your homework to find health care professionals who are on the cutting edge of the latest medical research and who will fully support you in the important and very personal decision you are making to carry a child and to breastfeed. Ask about any research studies at major health facilities in the area where you live—participating in any such study will help contribute much-needed information to researchers about pregnancy and cancer, and will also give you access to added care and medical expertise. And remember to draw upon the wonderful encouragement support groups can provide—join a breastfeeding support group and consider reconnecting with a breast cancer survivors group. No doubt the determination that brought you through your illness will make you doubly determined to breastfeed if you can. The breastfeeding bond between you, your baby, and your partner or spouse will be all the more precious for your efforts. We wish you the best!

BREAST AUGMENTATION, REDUCTION, OR MINOR BREAST SURGERY

If you've had surgery to enlarge or reduce the size of your breasts, your ability to breastfeed will depend upon how the surgery was done. Today, most surgeons are careful not to sever the milk ducts in the breast when performing any type of surgery to the breast. If the surgery was minor, such as removing a cyst or excising a benign lump, your breasts will probably be able to lactate. Breastfeeding after breast reduction surgery can be difficult because the surgery to reduce your breasts must preserve the duct system to the areola and nipple in order for you to be able to breastfeed. The duct system is not affected by augmentation surgery. However, the ability to breastfeed can be compromised by ruptured silicone implants and the effects of scar tissue in the breast, which can impede milk production. Breastfeeding when silicone implants are intact is considered safe; the implications of breastfeeding when silicone is known to be leaking from ruptured implants are unclear. If you've had silicone implants, your breast-milk should be examined by a laboratory for the presence of excessive amounts of silicone, which would indicate a ruptured implant, before you begin breastfeeding.

Each situation is unique, so if you have had breast surgery for any reason and want to breastfeed your baby, talk to your doctor. He or she can explain your medical condition and how it may or may not affect breastfeeding. If you are considering breast augmentation or reduction and plan to have more children and breastfeed in the future, be sure all medical practitioners involved are aware that you want to preserve your breastfeeding capability. Ask a lot of questions, and find out what your options are.

You're a Breastfeeding Family

Nursing might seem as if it involves a lot to remember at first, but with a little determination, you and your baby will be a happy and experienced nursing couple. And we haven't forgotten about you new fathers! The breastfeeding life has begun for the whole family. Whether you decide to breastfeed for two weeks, two months, or well through the "terrible twos," the breastfeeding relationship is an experience that will pass all too quickly. Before you know it, your "baby" will be asking you for the car keys! Revel in this time with your new baby and savor every moment. And even if friends and family encourage you with stories about their friend's sister's cousin's baby who was eating cheeseburgers at three months, remember that your baby doesn't need anything other than your breastmilk for the first six months of life. Give his system a chance to mature before exposing it to solids. You'll have plenty of time to experiment with new foods after six months, when your baby is meant to start trying gastronomical experimentation!

4

You're Really Doing It Now: The Breastfeeding Family in Action

The Nursing Personality

You and your baby are going with the flow (pun intended!) and nursing is fast becoming a part of your everyday life. By now you have gotten some clues about your baby's personality—and how that personality affects the breastfeeding relationship. Yes, *relationship!* The nursing relationship is the first interpersonal connection your baby will experience in life. As the two of you negotiate the ins and outs of nursing, you're probably eager to get some help in identifying specific "relationship" strategies that will help ensure breastfeeding success.

Take a look at the statements below, and check each one that applies to your baby's individual eating style. You may check off one statement or several. Then, read on to find the best ways to accommodate his breastfeeding M.O., what to watch out for, and how your own personality may match or clash with his feeding style.

☐ 1. You are all settled into your nursing haven with baby snuggled in your arms. You've got your herbal tea, you've got soft music cued up, and everything is set for the perfect nursing session—except your little one, who has fallen profoundly asleep before you've even unhooked your nursing bra.

☐ 2. The baby eats happily for ten minutes, and everything seems to be going fine. "I might even have time to cook a hot meal tonight," you think, until he spits his entire stomach contents onto your new white nursing shawl. You have to start all over again—and do another load of wash.

☐ 3. Your baby hasn't eaten for five hours, and although she doesn't seem hungry, you decide you should feed her. She has other plans. She nibbles at the breast for a minute or two, then prefers to play with the buttons on your shirt, watch her mobile, or gaze lovingly at your face. Nursing seems to be the last thing on her mind.

☐ 4. Your baby sucks intensely for five short minutes, then pushes away, ready to move on to the next exciting activity. He seems full and content, and you feel as if he has emptied one breast, but you wonder if he could possibly be finished already. Besides, you haven't even gotten a chance to relax!

☐ 5. After three or four minutes of nursing, the baby's eyelids begin to droop. A minute later, she has wandered off to dreamland. Your breast engorgement is only slightly relieved, and you know she hasn't filled her tummy, but she shows no signs of waking. One hour later (or even sooner), she's awake and ready for another round.

☐ 6. The baby loves to eat, but he also loves to coo, swipe, smile, giggle, kick, squirm, and stare. Nursing sessions seem to take forever because the baby sucks a little, laughs a little, squirms a little, then sucks a little more. He's eating, all right, but he seems to think you are an hors d'oeuvre tray in the middle of a cocktail party. An hour later, he's finally had his fill.

☐ 7. Your baby seems hungry all the time, but whenever she tries to eat, she breaks away again, cries a lot, and seems angry or upset. She used to eat well, but lately, you've noticed this increased fussiness and irritability.

☐ 8. Your baby eats and eats. He empties one breast, then the other, and keeps coming back for more. After an hour of nursing, you feel frustrated and drained (literally!). Will he ever give you a break?

☐ 9. You rarely have a problem with nursing. Whenever you nurse, the baby is game. She empties both breasts, burps politely, and moves on. And you thought breastfeeding would be difficult!

If you checked #1, you've got a Dozer. Your baby loves to sleep, at the expense of everything else. When you want to play, she's sleeping. When you want to show her off, she's sleeping. When you want to nurse, she's sound asleep. Should you wake her? In the first month or two, if she's gone for more than three or four hours without nursing, yes. But waking a soundly sleeping baby isn't as easy as you might think. Try positioning her in a sitting position, lightly tapping the bottom of her foot, or giving her a gentle facial massage. Talk to her in a cheerful, animated voice. When she starts to stir, step up your efforts until she looks at you. Tell her it's time to eat, then offer the breast. Chances are, she'll wake up enough to realize she's hungry, and be happy to oblige you.

Caution: If baby is very sluggish for more than a day or two and you can't get her to eat, call your doctor to rule out a health problem.

Mom's side: The Dozer is a difficult nursing type for energetic mothers who like to get things done. You might feel frustrated that she sleeps through everything. Don't worry—she isn't lazy. She's growing so quickly and experiencing so much that her body needs to replenish itself. Let her sleep. When she's two, you'll long for the days of the endless nap.

If you checked #2, you've got a Spit-Up Artist. Most babies spit up a little milk, especially when they haven't been burped sufficiently, but you might sometimes wonder why you bother feeding your baby at all, since the whole meal invariably comes back up in an impressive fountain of spit-up. Or, even if the baby keeps most of his dinner down at first, he may spit up just enough milk every hour or so to soil every piece of clothing both of you own on a daily basis. Some babies simply tend to spit up more than others, but if your baby's spitting up seems excessive, he may be eating too quickly. If he gulps frantically or chokes when you experience the milk ejection reflex, take him off the breast for a minute, express a little milk, then try again. Burping too roughly can also prompt a baby to lose his supper. If your baby is a Spit-Up Artist, handle him gently just before, during, and just after feeding. Sometimes merely propping him upright will elicit the necessary burps, whereas too much patting will bring up more than air. Keep him calm and still until he has a chance to digest his meal. And if he has literally lost his lunch, bite the bullet and nurse him again. Chances are, unless he's sick, he'll keep it down the second time.

Caution: If your baby spits up a very large amount after *every* meal, or projectile-vomits frequently, call your doctor, even if other signs of illness aren't present.

Mom's side: Squeamish and neatnik mothers have a hard time with Spit-Up Artists. Get used to keeping lots of spit-up rags handy (cloth diapers are great for this purpose), and for heaven's sake, don't wear your nicest clothes when nursing. Don't put your baby's nicest clothes on him, either, until you're sure his food is digested. Even then, be ready for surprises here and there. He can't help it. Some babies are just built that way.

If you checked #3, you've got a Browser. Your baby is interested in her world, and that's a good thing. She loves to look around, testing her environment, watching your face, and swiping at whatever seems to be in reach. The problem is, it's sometimes hard to convince her to get down to business and eat. Some babies just don't find nursing as interesting as looking around. To get her in the habit of regular meals she'll start and finish without intermissions, nurse her in an environment with as few distractions as possible. Turn the lights down low, don't play music, don't sit under interesting mobiles or dangly baby toys, and ask other family members to keep distractions to a minimum. Keep her eyes focused on your face, and keep encouraging her to nurse. She'll get the picture.

Caution: If your baby never seems hungry and refuses to eat, call your doctor to rule out a health problem.

Mom's side: The down-to-business mother may get frustrated by her Browser baby. Unfortunately, this may simply be a matter of differing personalities, and you, being the adult, must be the one to make allowances. Don't try to force your baby to adapt to a rigid schedule if it doesn't suit her. You can nudge her toward more consistent behavior, however, if you keep her schedule as regular as possible and encourage her to keep eating when she becomes distracted.

If you checked #4, you've got an Efficiency Expert. You have a tiny pro at your breast. He knows how to get the most out of nursing, extracting the maximum amount of milk in the minimum amount of time. He probably focuses well, and won't be easily distracted during nursing. By the same token, he won't want anyone bothering him, either, when he is concentrating on the business of his dinner. The Efficiency Expert may only nurse from one breast at each feeding, not wanting to waste time with two. You may need to feed him more often than the baby who nurses at both breasts and takes his time, but be reassured that your baby is getting a lot out of each nursing minute. Some efficiency experts can deftly drain a breast in five minutes.

FATHER ALERT!

DON'T FEEL LEFT OUT

It's true: the nursing relationship is a special exclusive bond between your partner and your child. But you have an important contribution you can make to your nursing couple. You can be the mediator, facilitator, and best friend, providing a shoulder to lean on and an ear to bend—for both of them! Encourage your partner to share with you the joys, frustrations, and challenges of breastfeeding—she'll appreciate a confidant who is nurturing and affectionate, a touchstone of nonjudgmental support and confidence-boosting. Your child, too, will love to confide in Dad—from cooing and gurgling to playing to fussing and crying, he'll love telling you all about it. Hold your nursing couple safe in your arms and let them know you are there for both of them.

Caution: Make sure your baby is gaining weight and has plenty of wet and soiled diapers. Some babies who only nurse for short periods aren't actually getting enough milk. Talk to your doctor if you are unsure.

Mom's side: The Efficiency Expert may be a challenge for the mother who likes to take her time, and especially the mother who looks forward to long, leisurely nursing sessions. If you find yourself disappointed that nursing is over so quickly, make up for it by adding extra cuddle time after nursing sessions. Hold your baby, talk to him, show him toys, and play games. Nursing isn't the only way to communicate physically with your child. If you are looking forward to the break, set aside as much time as you need, and don't let yourself leave your nursing haven until the time is up, even if the baby finished supping long before.

If you checked #5, you've got a Snacker-Snoozer. Like the Efficiency Expert, the Snacker-Snoozer's nursing sessions are often disappointingly short. The Snacker-Snoozer, however, usually doesn't get enough to eat before she falls peacefully asleep. She'd rather just wait until after her catnap for another snack. Unless you have nothing else to do but accommodate this kind of schedule, your job is to help keep the baby awake until she has nursed for at least ten or fifteen minutes. Try switching her from breast to breast whenever she starts to doze. Nurse her in an upright position, talk to her while nursing, lightly tap the bottoms of her feet, burp her, or change her diaper. If she snoozes despite your efforts, you may have to feed her more often for a few weeks until she gets more adept at staying awake. Keep up your efforts to teach her, gently, how to stay awake through dinner.

Caution: Make sure your little Snacker-Snoozer is getting enough milk. Watch for sufficient weight gain and lots of wet and soiled diapers. If you are worried your baby isn't eating enough and you are never able to keep her awake while nursing, talk to your doctor.

Mom's side: If you like to get things done and move on, or are impatient by nature, you may feel like you never get anywhere when it comes to your baby's nursing sessions. Every time you start, you have to stop, and before you can turn around, it's nursing time again. Remember that this pattern won't last. In the meantime, try to get things done in short spurts.

If you checked #6, you've got a Grazer. Like the Browser, the Grazer has a lot on his mind. Unlike the Browser, however, the Grazer relishes the whole nursing experience. That doesn't mean you should allow him to nurse all day long. The best way to help him focus on nursing is to feed him in a low-stimulus environment. Keep the lights down and distractions to a minimum. On the other hand, if you love to spend a long, leisurely hour nursing and snuggling, enjoy your little Grazer. All too soon, he'll be moving on to the high chair, the table, college . . . and you'll long for these affectionately unhurried meals.

Caution: Be sure not to rush the baby to finish so often that he never gets enough milk. Check with your doctor if you think the baby isn't gaining enough weight or if he isn't going through a lot of wet and soiled diapers each day.

Mom's side: Grazers are a real challenge to Type A personalities. "All right, already!" you may be dying to say. "Finish up and move on!" Remember that your Grazer is exploring the world in all its wonder, and when he does this while nursing, you get to be intimately involved. Your baby is challenging you to slow down and smell the flowers. Not a bad idea.

If you checked #7, you've got a Fussy Feeder. Your baby may want everything to be just right before she can really settle in for a good meal—her position, her clothing, *your* position may all need to be adjusted until you find the perfect fit. On the other hand, sometimes fussiness occurs suddenly, in which case you'll want to look for potential problems. Consider your diet. Have you recently started eating something new that might be affecting the taste of your breastmilk, such as broccoli, chocolate, spicy foods, or coffee? Have you recently become tense or is your family experiencing any new stress? Have you moved recently, changed the baby's sleeping arrangements, or brought a new pet into the home? Have you or has anyone else in the house been sick? All these factors can affect a sensitive baby's appetite and/or nursing comfort level. Try to remedy any possible stressors and your baby will probably fall back into her normal eating pattern.

Caution: If your baby shows signs of stress or pain and you can't determine the cause (or even if you can), talk to your pediatrician.

Mom's side: It can be very frustrating to have an irritable baby, especially when her irritation keeps her from getting the sustenance you know she needs. Remember that the more frustrated you get, however, the more stressed your baby will become. Babies are very in-tune with their mothers, so some major stress management may be in order if you want to get back in synch with your baby and reassure her that all is well with her world (see chapter 7).

If you checked #8, you've got an Eager Eater. This baby loves nursing. I mean, he *really* loves nursing. If your baby wants to nurse all the time, even after your breasts are drained, you may find yourself with several problems. You may experience more severe nipple irritation than other moms. You may find you actually have no time for anything else at all. You may feel resentful toward your baby for being so demanding. And your milk supply may increase so much that you feel constantly engorged when you aren't nursing. The Eager Eater doesn't actually need to eat all the time, but he does seem to have more intense sucking needs than other babies. Maybe you are adamantly against the pacifier, but guess what? In your case, it just may preserve your sanity. If you take the pacifier away at three to six months, your baby won't be too attached yet, and you won't have to worry about having a grade-schooler who still walks around with "the plug." But to get you through these first few months, consider it, unless you'd rather just strap him to your chest with a sling and let him nurse as he likes (some women find this a pleasant option).

Caution: It's extremely rare for a breastfeeding baby to become overweight (a condition more often associated with formula-fed babies), but if your baby eats constantly and seems to be getting very large, check with your doctor to make sure he isn't overweight.

Mom's side: If the twenty-four-hour-a-day milk bank just isn't your style and you feel you really do need a break from your Eager Eater, don't feel bad about pumping breastmilk (See "Breast Pump Choices" later in this chapter) and letting your partner take on a few feedings with the bottle after nursing is well established, or even resorting to an occasional bottle of formula if you are truly tapped out.

If you checked #9, you've got a Nursing Angel. Count your blessings; you're a lucky mother, indeed!

THERE IS A WORLD OUT THERE: GOING OUT WITH YOUR BABY

Obviously, you can't stay in forever. Eventually you're going to have to leave the comfortable and safe shelter of your home to buy groceries, see friends, or just remind yourself that there is a world out there. You'll probably stay mostly housebound for the first few weeks, but when you do venture out, your baby will want to be with you. Assuming she is in good health, she can make social calls and "help you" with errands at as young as two or three weeks (check with your doctor about how long he or she recommends you wait before taking your infant out). You can leave the baby with a sitter occasionally, but most of the time you'll want to pack her up and bring her along. She wants to be with you, she'll need to nurse, and she wants to see that there is a world out there, too. The change of scenery will probably interest her.

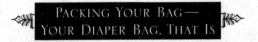

PACKING YOUR BAG— YOUR DIAPER BAG. THAT IS

Going out isn't what it used to be before your "baby makes three" days. You can't just grab your purse and car keys. Your baby has a few supplies he needs, too, and forgetting anything important can mean disaster or, at least, severe inconvenience. Your main ally against distress is a well-equipped diaper bag. Buy one that is roomy but not too bulky, with lots of pockets and a changing pad. The bag should be washable or wipeable, with a sturdy strap so you can carry it over your shoulder and still have your hands free.

Here's what you'll need to put in it:

◎ At least ten diapers—kept in the bag at all times (you never know how long you'll be out)

◎ A good supply of diaper wipes—they come in portable packages that are easy to carry (also great for cleaning up sticky hands and faces, or washing your own hands after a diaper change)

◎ At least five spit-up rags (cloth diapers work great for this purpose)

◎ Infant Tylenol (acetaminophen) (Helpful to have with you after your child receives certain vaccinations, if the pediatrician recommends it; also, you never know when you might need to bring down a fever. Remember, too, children under fifteen should not take aspirin, as it has been linked to a rare but serious disorder called Reye's syndrome. Physicians recommend acetaminophen instead of aspirin for infants and children.)

◎ A mercury thermometer

◎ K-Y Jelly (for use with thermometers when taking an infant's rectal temperature)

◎ Two outfit changes (spit-up is notorious for ruining the cutest ensemble just before anyone sees it!)

◎ A couple of pairs of socks or booties

◎ A receiving blanket or two (for when it gets unexpectedly cold, or the baby needs extra security, or to facilitate subtle nursing in public)

◎ A rattle or other small, amusing toys

◎ A front-pack infant carrier or sling (excellent to have when you need your hands free, and for nursing)

Sound like a lot? It is, but if you keep the diaper bag stocked, going out isn't a bother. In fact, it can be fun. And, hey, bottle-fed babies require even more stuff!

SENSORY OVERLOAD

Your baby isn't used to a lot of sensory stimulation, especially at first. He's been safely enclosed in a dark, insulated place where sound is muted and movement is cushioned. Many babies find outings stimulating, but even the most curious will eventually get his fill. For some, it doesn't take long at all. Pay attention to your baby when you are out, or whenever you alter his routine. If he starts to cry for no apparent reason, won't look you in the eye, looks scared or unusually wide-eyed, falls asleep when it isn't his normal nap time, or acts otherwise distraught, he has probably had enough. Take him to a quiet place, drape a blanket over him (or put him under a maternity shirt or trapeze-style top), and nurse. Nursing is a great way for babies to temporarily tune out an overstimulating environment and concentrate on something calming, familiar, and safe. If your baby seems particularly sensitive, try to limit outings for the first month or two. This is preferable to leaving him with a sitter. Staying at home without you in these early weeks will probably be more stressful to him than leaving home with you. After all, to your newborn, "home" means "with Mom."

NURSING IN PUBLIC

If you are planning to be out for more than an hour or two, you will probably need to nurse your baby. Many new mothers are self-conscious about nursing in public, and although response to this issue is becoming more positive, some people (usually people without children) are still uncomfortable being around a mother who is nursing. However, it is your legal right to breastfeed your baby anywhere you are allowed to be with your baby, and many states have been legally redefining the law specifically to include tolerance and encouragement of breastfeeding mothers. In fact, as of July 1, 1996, twelve states (Florida, Illinois, Idaho, Iowa, Michigan, New York, Nevada, North Carolina, Texas, Utah, Virginia,

OTHER THINGS TO REMEMBER ON AN OUTING

◎ The stroller. The type that can accommodate a car seat/infant carrier are handy, but be careful you don't keep your baby strapped in the same infant carrier all day long just because it is so convenient.

◎ Wear something nursing-friendly.

◎ Always double-check that the car seat is buckled in, and that she is strapped in correctly.

◎ In the midst of all the fuss, don't forget the baby! (It has happened.)

and Wisconsin) have passed legislation directly addressing breastfeeding legal issues, all in favor of breastfeeding rights. Some laws clearly state that breastfeeding can in no way be interpreted as indecent exposure, even if a woman's nipple is exposed during or incidental to breastfeeding. Other states have proclaimed that breastfeeding mothers be released from jury duty when such service would keep her from breastfeeding (even in states without this ruling, a breastfeeding mother can appear before the judge and request an exemption). Many states include verbiage stating that breastfeeding is an important act of nurturing and nourishing a child and that breastfeeding must be encouraged.

More and more businesses are facilitating breastfeeding as they become aware that customers need this service, and it is highly unlikely that anyone could charge you for indecent exposure and win. If someone ever asks you to stop nursing in public (this occasionally happens to new mothers who are still getting used to nursing and therefore may appear more conspicuous), you may want to inform the person, calmly and confidently, that you have a legal right to breastfeed.

Be aware, however, that your right to breastfeed may not extend to *every* situation; you may not be able to leave your job on a daily basis to nurse if leaving your job site is not generally allowed. In addition, you may not be able to bring your child to your job to nurse if bringing children to your job isn't generally allowed. In *Dike* v. *Orange County School Board* in 1981, the U.S. Court of Appeals ruled that mothers have a constitutional right to breastfeed, but did not support the subject of the case— a teacher who wanted to nurse her baby on her lunch break and was not allowed to do so because of school rules prohibiting teachers from leaving the school during the day. In other words, state laws or other rules made for other purposes may stand if you try to be excepted for the purpose of breastfeeding.

If you find yourself in the company of people who simply are *uncomfortable* with what you and your baby are doing, you can handle it in one of two ways: You can feed your baby anyway and let the others deal with it. (After all, if you don't breastfeed in front of others, people's attitudes will never become more informed.) Or, if it bothers *you* that someone else is bothered, be discreet. You can either excuse yourself to a more secluded location (a bathroom, an unoccupied bedroom if you are visiting someone's home, or even an isolated corner; many stores will allow you to use their dressing rooms if you ask), or you can drape a receiving blanket over your infant, or even nurse him under your shirt if it is large enough. If your baby is feeling overstimulated, he will probably love nursing under such a protective cover, and unless you tell people what you are doing, many will think you are just holding a sleeping baby. Mothers have been known to nurse this way in every imaginable public place, including parks, restaurants, schools, malls, and airplanes (nursing has the added benefit of relieving pressure in a baby's ears at takeoff and landing, although you may want to keep your baby in his

FATHER ALERT!

CROWD CONTROL, GOFER, DEFENDER OF THE BREAST!

Packing up the baby and venturing out in public with your newly expanded family can make a trip to the grocery store a tour de force. Suddenly, the world seems full of obstacles and threats you hadn't perceived before. Your partner will be doing everything she can to keep your baby protected and well nourished en route, but on family outings, you can do a lot to help them both from becoming overwhelmed.

In crowded environments or in situations where lots of friends want to see your new child, you can direct traffic, clear the way, or organize a "one-at-a-time" system for greeting him. If he needs to nurse, help your partner seek out an appropriate, relatively quiet spot. If your partner is ever criticized or reprimanded for breastfeeding in public, you can be her champion, calmly and firmly informing the ignorant critic of a nursing mother's legal rights. You can also help out by running errands and accomplishing everyday tasks outside the home, which might take twice as long now with a baby in tow.

infant seat when traveling by air). Most important, don't let other people's attitudes keep you from doing what you know is right for your baby and for your family.

RULES FOR SUCCESSFUL OUTINGS

When you plan outings with your baby, awareness of a few basics will make the experiences happier for everyone:

Don't plan too much at once, especially at first. You may have a list of a hundred things that need to be done, but you will be more productive if you space your errands out between several trips. A baby gets cranky if she is continually carted from place to place and transferred relentlessly from car seat to stroller to car seat to stroller without a chance to relax, nurse, and nap. When she's had enough, she'll let you know. Trying to finish your last seven errands while she is wailing miserably is virtually impossible. If you can't go home when she is worn out, at least park the car, take her out of her car seat, lavish her with touch and attention, and nurse her awhile. If you're lucky, she'll go to sleep, but she may cry all the way home. You may have to stop on the side of a quiet street (don't pick a busy road, for obvious reasons) or in a parking lot to nurse. If you plan your outings to be brief, you'll avoid the misery of being caught in traffic, unable to hold and calm your exhausted child. Next time, you'll know how long she is likely to last.

Don't forget to wear something nursing-friendly. If you find yourself in a public place and your baby is frantic to nurse, you won't want to pull down the whole top of that cute sundress or lift that entire jumper over him. The easiest ensemble is a maternity or trapeze-style top with shorts or leggings, or a roomy shirt or dress with buttons and a receiving blanket for any necessary cover-up.

Don't expose your baby to unhealthy environments. Smoky restaurants, extra-crowded or especially loud events, such as concerts or festivals, places where lots of people have been drinking and may lack judgment, or any other place where the environment may be unhealthy, uncontrolled, or dangerous, are best left for grown-ups. Use your good judgment.

Beware of the hot seat. Don't deposit a child in her car seat after the car has been sitting in the sun until you first feel the seat. Car seats can become red hot and can burn a baby. Especially check metal and plastic buckles.

Play germ shield. One of the more fun aspects of an outing with your baby is the continual praise you'll both receive. "He's so cute!" "Look at her darling outfit!" "He's so big for three months!" "Look at those beautiful eyes!" Mothers live for this kind of thing, so the last thing you will want to do to a kindly and well-meaning stranger is snap, "Don't touch her!" However, babies are very susceptible to germs (although the nursing baby is much less so). A pat on the head probably won't hurt your newborn, but if strangers or even friends want to kiss or hold the baby, or if someone has had any kind of illness, such as a cold or flu, kindly ask that they keep their distance. Anyone who touches a newborn should wash his or her hands first (even you!). Small children, who are particularly fascinated with babies, are notorious for carrying cold and flu germs, and will often put their hands or mouths all over your baby before you even know they are there, so be on your guard in public places with a lot of kids, such as parks, malls, grocery stores, and airports. If you are uncomfortable with anyone touching or holding your baby, speak up! Your newborn is too little to defend herself—that's your job! Don't let the fear of offending someone keep you from protecting her rights. (And while you're at it, remember to teach your own young children never to touch anyone's baby without first asking the parents' permission.)

Before long, your new family will be a traveling team. Practice makes perfect. More than anything else, remember that your baby wants to be near you and needs your touch. No matter where you are, make sure she knows you and your spouse or partner are close by and ready to meet her needs.

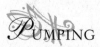

PUMPING

Yes, there *are* going to be some times when you won't be able to nurse your baby—no matter how diligently you try to be there for every feeding. It's O.K.! You may have multiples and you need a break (or you don't have multiples and you need a break!); maybe you have an all-important errand out of the house, such as a freelance work assignment that has to be delivered to a client—without a baby in tow; perhaps you just need an uninterrupted night's sleep and your partner agrees to administer the two A.M. feeding; or you could be planning a romantic dinner out while the grandparents watch over your little one for a couple of hours. Whatever the reason, don't feel guilty about leaving an expressed bottle of breastmilk for a sitter to feed to your baby. (But don't offer your baby a bottle for the first two or three weeks of life, until nursing is well established.) And consider this: if you return to work after maternity leave and want to continue breastfeeding, the breast pump will become an invaluable—and necessary—tool. (See chapter 9 for more on breastfeeding after returning to the office.) A breast pump is much more effective at extracting larger quantities of milk than expressing by hand (see "Expressing Breastmilk Manually" on page 56); manual expression is best left for tasks such as relieving engorgement or to entice an infant to nurse with a few drops of expressed milk.

Pumping might seem like a lot of trouble, but once you are used to it, it is not too much more trouble than buying and preparing formula, with one crucial, added benefit: your baby will only be drinking breastmilk. Even if she is drinking from a bottle, if that bottle contains your milk, it is still tailor-made for her, and filled with the superior nutrition and immune-boosting ingredients not present in formula. Finding a good quality breast pump is half the battle.

Before you begin your pumping session, make sure your hands are clean; wash them with disinfectant soap and scrub under your nails with a brush. Drink a glass of fluid or have some hot soup. Get comfortable. Take a few deep breaths, then follow the directions for your individual pump. Many women find it difficult to trigger a milk ejection reflex when her baby isn't around. If, for some reason, you can't be with him while you are express-

(Relatively) Polite Ways to Keep People from Pawing

◉ "If you don't mind, the baby has had a little cold, so please just look."

◉ "I'm sorry, but I have this 'Wash Your Hands First' rule. I know you understand!"

◉ "I'm such a protective mother, but have you been around anyone with a cold?"

◉ "I assume you haven't been sick? I'm extra careful since it's that season, you know!"

◉ "Isn't she cute? When she's a little older, you'll be able to hold her!"

◉ "I'd hate for your child to catch something; could you keep him back just a bit?"

◉ "Look, but please don't touch." (Spoken with a winning smile, of course!)

ing milk, keep a photograph of him nearby. Hold it and study it. Imagine him crying. Imagine nursing him. This really works! Your mind is powerful, and the thought of your baby is often all it takes. The more you pump, the easier it will be, just like nursing, so don't give up after just a few tries.

If you are expressing milk to be fed to your baby more than thirty minutes after you've pumped it, put the milk in the refrigerator or store it in the freezer. Store the milk in clean, heavy-duty

BREAST PUMP CHOICES

Several types of breast pumps are on the market. Choosing which one to buy will depend on how often you plan to pump, how much time you will have, and how much money you want to spend. Talk to a certified lactation consultant or call your local La Leche League for information on the pumps currently available, which pumps they recommend, and the best way to acquire one, such as local places to rent or purchase.

Manual pumps. These pumps have no motor and are inexpensive but not very efficient. Several types include bulb pumps, trigger-operated pumps, syringe pumps, and convertible pumps (which can be plugged in or operated manually). Manual pumps take some strength and a lot more time. They are conveniently portable, but not good for regular, daily pumping. They are more suited for relieving occasional engorgement. They can sometimes be slightly painful and harsh on the nipples.

Battery-operated pumps. These pumps are inexpensive compared to electric pumps, and also very portable, but they use up batteries quickly. Some people swear by these pumps, but they are slower than electric and not extremely practical for regular, frequent use. Some also plug in, but aren't hands-free like the more expensive electric models. They work great when you are experiencing the milk ejection reflex, but that can be hard to trigger when your baby is nowhere in sight.

Electric pumps. These pumps are fast and efficient. Some empty both breasts at once. Others leave one breast free, and if you nurse the baby on one breast while pumping the other breast, pumping becomes even more efficient because the milk ejection reflex comes easily. Electric pumps don't require any kind of manual operation and don't need to be held while pumping, so your hands are free. They are expensive, however, and not very portable. Hospitals or other local sources may rent electric pumps, or consider purchasing one in conjunction with other nursing mothers, to lower the cost to each.

freezer bags or in sterilized plastic nursing bottles. (Don't use glass bottles—certain important white blood cells in mother's milk can stick to glass.) If you've only been able to express an ounce or two, you can still freeze the milk and add more to the same container later. But never add warm milk to frozen milk—chill milk for several hours in the refrigerator before adding to a container of frozen milk (so the frozen milk doesn't thaw at all).

Thaw frozen bottles or bags by running warm water over them or using a bottle warmer. Do not microwave breastmilk. The microwave process destroys certain important components of the milk; it can also heat the milk unevenly, which may put the baby at risk for burns. Do not heat milk in a pan on the stove, either, which can cause it to curdle. Milk need only be room temperature or slightly warmer for feeding. After breastmilk is thawed, use it within half an hour. Freshly pumped breastmilk will stay good in the refrigerator for twenty-four hours, in the freezer for six months. Once a baby has introduced saliva by sucking on a bottle of milk, the leftover amount must be discarded. Bacteria grow exceptionally fast in breastmilk.

If you need to travel with a bottle of expressed breastmilk for any reason, keep the milk as cold as possible. Put it in a thermos or an insulated cold pack or cooler (you can buy small, portable coolers made specifically for keeping breastmilk cold).

You might be reluctant to pump at first because it feels so unnatural. Granted, it is. You might feel like a dairy cow hooked up to a milking machine, and you might be self-conscious about how ridiculous it looks. Just remember that you are doing it for your baby. Remember how much better breastmilk is for her. That said, if you try and try and it just doesn't work for you or you just can't make yourself comfortable with the process, an occasional formula feeding isn't going to hurt. Don't feel guilty. Do what you need to do to be a good, relaxed, happy mother.

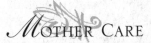

MOTHER CARE

In the midst of all these changes, don't forget to take care of *yourself*. You are important, and your baby's well-being depends on *your* well-being, so keep yourself healthy, relax, and try not to let the barrage of visitors, the demands of family, and the seemingly endless obligations of newborn care overwhelm you (easier said than done). Most importantly, remember the Ten Commandments of New Mother Care. Memorize them. Live them. You'll thank yourself later.

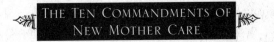

THE TEN COMMANDMENTS OF NEW MOTHER CARE

I. Thou Shalt Sleep. "Sleep?" you say, with a hysterical giggle. "What's sleep?" You *can* get enough sleep. Let the baby sleep with you. During the day, nap when your child naps. Let the housework go for a while. Order out for dinner (something healthy—a gourmet veggie pizza with whole wheat crust, Thai food, turkey sub sandwiches), or send Dad out for a big bag of premixed salad and a selection of precut veggies. Whatever it takes to squeeze in a nap, do it. You need to be alert and your body will be more resistant to sickness and emotional upheaval when you are well rested (see chapter 7 for more on stress and the breastfeeding relationship).

II. Thou Shalt Not Be Afraid to Ask for Help. Remember that guy who helped make this baby? He'll probably do a lot for you if you just ask him. He may not know what you need unless you tell him. Don't fall into the "only I can do it right" trap. You may even discover that he has a *better* way of handling certain things. If you are feeling emotional and judgmental, try your hardest not to criticize Dad's efforts to help you. Praise will be more likely to ensure continued support and increased domestic confidence (unless you are already married to SuperDad, in which case you can disregard all suggestions for easing him into a more domestic role). If friends or relatives offer to come over, cook a meal, clean up, or watch the baby for a few hours, *let them!* Give yourself a break.

III. Thou Shalt Continue to Take Thy Prenatal Vitamins. Even though you are no longer pregnant, you are still nutritionally supporting your baby. You probably won't always have time to eat everything you need every day, and vitamins are a good insurance policy. Support your body's maintenance efforts. Remember, though, that taking megadoses of vitamins may be harmful; consult your physician about the right supplement dosage for your individual needs. (For more on vitamins and supplements, see page 109.)

IV. Thou Shalt Stay Nourished and Hydrated. To keep your strength and your mood up, keep eating. Make every bite nutritious and energizing. Think nutrient-dense rather than low-cal (for example, choose small amounts of dried fruit, almonds, or egg salad over large quantities of popcorn, pretzels, and so-called diet foods). Snack frequently on healthy food like raw veggies, seasonal fruit, dried apricots, yogurt, tuna, whole wheat crackers, and peanut, almond, or sesame butter. Keep a gallon jug of water in the refrigerator or on the counter and refill your glass throughout the day. Try to go through a gallon every two days or so. (For lots more on nutrition and breastfeeding, see chapter 5.)

V. Thou Shalt Not Chide Thyself for Feeling Emotional. It will probably happen: a sudden outburst of tears for no reason, a pervasive melancholy about your "lost life," a frustrated outburst at your uncooperative partner, uncontrollable sobbing at the emotional intensity of anything on TV having to do with a mother and a baby. Don't worry. You can't help it. Your hormones are running amuck! They'll stabilize in a week or two. *However,* if you feel seriously depressed to the point that you have difficulty functioning or caring for your baby, or if you experience feelings of violence or have irrational thoughts, call your doctor immediately. Postpartum depression and even postpartum psychosis do occur in many new moms, up to several years after a baby's birth, and are easily treatable.

VI. Thou Shalt Reflect on Thine Own Parents. Think about it— your parents experienced everything you are now experiencing, and *you* were the baby that engendered the same intense feelings in your parents that your baby has prompted you to feel. Suddenly, your parents' behavior over the years may make a little more sense to you. This will happen more and more often, and although you will not become your parents (no, really, you won't, although the resemblance may become more striking), you may be able to understand them in a way you never could have if you hadn't had your own child. Communicate with your parents as much as possible if they live far away. Let them in on your new understanding. On the other hand, remember this is *your* baby, not theirs. You and your partner are the parents now, and you make the rules. Understand your parents, appreciate their feelings, but don't let them bully you. You have moved to a new dimension in the parent-child relationship. Try your best to keep the lines of communication open, affectionate, and mature.

If one or both of your parents (or in-laws!) have come to stay with you, to help out in the early weeks, you may have mixed feelings. You will be thankful for the help; on the other hand, if they tend to offer a lot of unsolicited advice or try to take over the baby, you may also feel resentment. Some new grandparents are wonderful at stepping back and letting the new parents take the lead, offering advice only when it is requested and helping only where help is desired. New grandparents are only human, however. They have had years of parenting experience, and may find the temptation to lecture you irresistible. Remember that you will always be their baby, and they want to help you, which for some parents means shielding you from what they perceive as mistakes. Again, the best way to keep everyone friendly is to keep communicating. If your mother is driving you crazy (for example), remind her, nicely, that you are the mom now. She may enjoy her new grandchild, and you appreciate her help, but she has to follow the rules you and your partner have established for your family. Making your visiting parents feel invaluable while at the same time enforcing your own authority is a tricky but crucial balance you'll need to explore one day at a time.

Another important consideration is the possibility that parental help may be appreciated by you but not your partner, or vice versa. Above all, do not let new grandparents interfere with your relationship. If one of you has a problem with the temporary situation, you must make it known to the other. Together, you can figure out a way to make things work.

VII. Thou Shalt Devote Time Every Day Exclusively to Thyself.
You will need time every day away from your partner, the baby, and all responsibility, to do nothing other than relax and think about your new life. Let your partner take over, even for a quick fifteen minutes. Go someplace quiet, close the door, relax, breathe deeply, enjoy a warm or a cool drink, close your eyes, and remember that being a mother is a wonderful new part of yourself—but not the only part! Reconnect with yourself as often as you can.

VIII. Thou Shalt Maintain Thy Personal Hygiene. This, believe it or not, is far easier said than done. Days will slip by more quickly than you can imagine, and you will realize you haven't showered, your hair is a mess, and you are wearing clothes covered in baby spit-up. Also, believe it or not, you probably won't care very much, especially not at first, but you owe it to yourself (not to anyone else) to keep yourself feeling refreshed, clean, and able to face the world, whenever it may come knocking unexpectedly. Don't try to look like you are ready to go to the office. You needn't even get dressed, but a shower or bath and a change of clothes, a healthy teeth brushing, flossing, hair combing, and face scrub every day will energize you and make you feel good about yourself, despite the extra pounds you may still be carrying, the hair loss you may suddenly be experiencing, or the stretch marks you may be sporting. (You can deal with those later.)

IX. Thou Shalt Touch and Be Touched. Touching and being touched are important for maintaining the sense of well-being in all humans. Don't let one single day go by without touching, hugging, and kissing your partner, even though it may be too soon to resume sexual relations. Once you are ready for sex, don't delay. Your relationship with your partner needs this physical and emotional connection to help sustain it during the difficult transition to parenthood. Also, even when you aren't breastfeeding, touch, hold, and hug your baby as much as possible, and don't forget to stay in physical contact with other children in the family who may be feeling a little neglected these days.

X. Thou Shalt Breathe Fresh Air and Bathe in Sunshine. Every day (weather permitting—spare yourself and your baby if it is very hot or bitterly cold), for your own sake and the sake of your baby, go for a walk in the sunshine. In summer, mornings or late afternoons are best, in order to avoid the extreme heat and harmful sun rays. In winter, venture out during the middle of the day when temperatures are at their peak. Inhale deeply and let the sun shine on your face and arms. Walk briskly, for a pleasant cardiovascular and muscular workout. Look around you and enjoy your surroundings. Point things out to your baby. Breathe. The more family members who are able to join you on walks, the better. Walking will help to melt those extra pounds away, and help your muscles remember how to work, too. (See the section on exercise in chapter 7 for more benefits.)

FATHER ALERT!

THE TEN COMMANDMENTS OF NEW FATHER CARE

Yes, new fathers, we have some commandments for you, too!

I. Thou Shalt Not Feel Guilty for Wanting to Get Out of the House. Your partner will understand if you give yourself an occasional break. Go for a drive, a walk, meet a friend, or just retire to an out-of-the-way place at home, close the door, and relax for a while. Then offer to give *her* a break!

II. Thou Shalt Request Time Alone with Thy Partner. Your partner may be so involved with the baby that she, understandably, forgets to make time for the two of you. This "couple time" is important for a healthy family, however, so remind her. You should spend at least thirty minutes every day alone together.

III. Thou Shalt Have Sex. After the doctor gives the O.K., approach your partner about resuming sexual relations. Many new fathers are reluctant to suggest this step, but chances are, your partner is either ready, or ready to have you help her get ready (see the section on sex in chapter 8 for an explanation of why some women may need a little encouragement when it comes to postpartum sex, and how you can help).

IV. Thou Shalt Acknowledge the Depths of Thine Emotion.
You have helped to create a life and you may be overwhelmed at the love you feel for that tiny person. Perhaps
you are hesitant to let yourself feel that love because of its
intensity. Part of effective fathering is surrendering yourself
to that huge, indescribable feeling. Let yourself feel your
protective instincts, your nurturing instincts, your tenderness, and your love. And don't worry—if you don't feel it
yet, you will.

V. Thou Shalt Freely Boast about Thy Progeny. You deserve
to brag. Carry a picture of your baby, and show it to everyone. Of course, you'll want to exercise a degree of discretion
at your workplace, but even there, people will probably
want to see a picture, at least once!

VI. Thou Shalt Practice Baby Care and Enjoy the Benefits.
Changing that smelly, gooey diaper probably doesn't seem
appealing (it's no picnic for your partner, either). Maybe
bathing that tiny, fragile baby seems too risky. Perhaps you
think baby care is best left to the mother, at least at first.
Wrong! The only way you will become comfortable about
baby care, let alone with your new child, is to practice. You
will probably do things a little differently than your partner,
but that's fine. Every parent has his or her unique style. If
you have a question, ask, but don't be afraid to meet your
baby's needs. The reward is a feeling of involvement in your
family, and a more intimate physical and emotional relationship with your child. Fathering only begins with diapers,
baths, and peek-a-boo. It quickly grows into something
indescribably wonderful. Start that relationship growing
right at the start.

**VII. Thou Shalt Not Allow Others to Come between You and
Your Partner.** New parents are usually bombarded with unsolicited advice and interference by friends and relatives alike. If

in-laws, best friends, coworkers, or anyone else is coming between you and your partner, causing disagreements or unhappiness, make a pact with your partner that family comes first, and although you don't have to be rude or unkind to others, the opinions and influences of others must remain secondary to your new family.

VIII. Thou Shalt Not Sacrifice Thy Health. Through sleepless nights and frantic mealtimes, make a concerted effort to eat healthy foods, avoid health-destroying habits like smoking and drinking, exercise regularly (even if it only means a brisk walk with the baby in the stroller), and practice stress management (see chapter 7 for techniques). A healthy dad handles fatherhood far better than a sick, out-of-shape, or stressed-out dad.

IX. Thou Shalt Acknowledge Thy Negative Feelings. Maybe you are intensely jealous of the close relationship between mother and baby. Maybe you are jealous of the time she spends with the new child—time that used to be spent with you. Maybe ever since you saw her giving birth, you are having a problem seeing your partner in a sexual way. Maybe you find breastfeeding uncomfortably sexual or strange, even though you know it is better for your baby. Maybe you are disturbed by your partner's breasts leaking milk. Maybe you are angry at being left out of the parenting experience. All these feelings are natural and common. Parenting is difficult, especially when you are new at it. Plus, pregnancy and childbirth sent hormones coursing through your partner which triggered an intense maternal instinct. You, on the other hand, were an observer throughout the pregnancy, and now are suddenly expected to adapt to fatherhood. No wonder your emotions are mixed!

Whatever your feelings, talk about them with your partner. Chances are, she has a few fears also, and talking will probably make you both feel better. If your feelings truly disturb you or you aren't able to talk to your partner about them, talk to a friend or call a counselor. You don't have to feel badly, and you shouldn't let your fear of expressing your emotions potentially harm your relationship with your partner or your baby.

X. Love Thy Child with All Thy Heart, with All Thy Soul, and with All Thy Mind. No love is more powerful than the love of a parent for a child. Revel in it and you will feel as if the universe has given you a spectacular gift—because it has.

5

◂ Feeding the Family

What a Nursing Mom Should Eat

Beyond simply eating a balanced diet, the nursing mother has special nutritional needs. The good part is that nursing allows you to eat an extra five hundred calories (approximately) beyond what it takes to maintain your prepregnancy weight. (Some sources quote more, but you built up extra fat while pregnant to burn while nursing, so you want to use it.) New mothers rarely have time to count calories, however. A less obsessive and easier way to gauge your progress is to weigh yourself once a week at the same time (say, every Sunday morning). Don't worry about losing any weight for the first six weeks. You probably dropped quite a bit of weight (baby, fluid, etc.) in the first couple of weeks, and now your body needs to adjust and heal. After six weeks, if you gradually lose weight at the approximate rate of one pound per week until you reach your prepregnancy weight (or your ideal weight, if you were a bit high or low when you became pregnant), you are doing well.

If you are gaining weight postdelivery, you are eating too much. Cut back on empty calories! Get used to stopping before you are full. Try to eat smaller amounts of food at

STAY OUT OF THE FAST LANE

Losing weight too quickly releases toxins stored in fat cells into breastmilk—so does fasting. Many people enjoy fasting as a way to cleanse and purify the system, rest the digestive tract, and generally purge themselves of impurities. This is fine for the autonomous adult, but the breastfeeding mother is not autonomous. Those impurities you are purging will go straight into your breastmilk and into your baby. It isn't worth the risk. If you enjoy fasting, wait to resume this practice until after you have weaned your baby.

each meal. Smaller meals are easier on your digestion; you'll feel lighter and more energetic.

THE FOOD PYRAMID FOR NURSING MOTHERS

If you are looking for structure in your diet, the following is a basic guideline for your nutritional requirements based on the USDA Food Pyramid principle, which has officially replaced the famous "Four Food Groups" as the healthy way to eat, according to the USDA recommendation. The pyramid below is specially tailored for the nursing mother. Use common sense regarding what food belongs in each category if what you want to eat isn't listed.

The Food Pyramid principle is simple. Eat most of what is on the bottom, eat least of what is on the top. Numbers of servings are approximate and meant to be a guide. A serving in the grain group is the approximate equivalent of one slice of bread or one-half cup of cooked grains, corn, or peas. A vegetable serving and a fruit serving are both one-half cup cooked, one cup raw, or one medium piece. Approximately three ounces of meat or fish

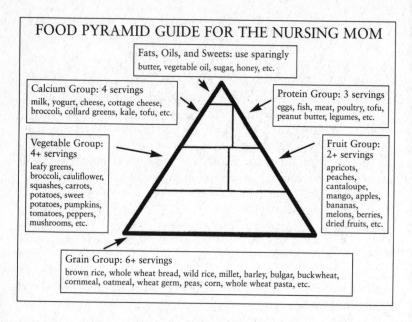

FOOD PYRAMID GUIDE FOR THE NURSING MOM

Fats, Oils, and Sweets: use sparingly
butter, vegetable oil, sugar, honey, etc.

Calcium Group: 4 servings
milk, yogurt, cheese, cottage cheese,
broccoli, collard greens, kale, tofu, etc.

Protein Group: 3 servings
eggs, fish, meat, poultry, tofu,
peanut butter, legumes, etc.

Vegetable Group: 4+ servings
leafy greens, broccoli, cauliflower, squashes, carrots, potatoes, sweet potatoes, pumpkins, tomatoes, peppers, mushrooms, etc.

Fruit Group: 2+ servings
apricots, peaches, cantaloupe, mango, apples, bananas, melons, berries, dried fruits, etc.

Grain Group: 6+ servings
brown rice, whole wheat bread, wild rice, millet, barley, bulgar, buckwheat, cornmeal, oatmeal, wheat germ, peas, corn, whole wheat pasta, etc.

THE LIGHT AND DARK SIDE OF RICE

Rice is a nutritious, easy-to-prepare food, but not all rice is created equal. Although nonfat and more nutritious than many processed foods, white rice has the bran and germ removed. The bran and germ contain valuable vitamins and minerals, amino acids, and fiber. Brown rice retains the bran and germ, and so has a good ratio of all the basic nutrients. White rice, in comparison, is nutritionally deficient, so choose brown when you have the choice.

Although raw white rice can be stored at room temperature almost indefinitely, brown rice should only be stored for six months because the oil in the bran can go rancid. Or, store raw brown rice in the refrigerator or freezer.

comprises a serving, as does one-half cup of legumes, about three tablespoons peanut butter, or one egg. A serving of dairy equals one cup of milk or yogurt, three-quarters cup cottage cheese, or about one ounce of hard cheese.

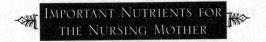

IMPORTANT NUTRIENTS FOR THE NURSING MOTHER

When you were pregnant, it was important to get adequate protein for baby building. Now, you should cut back a bit on the protein and concentrate on calcium, which will aid in milk production and possibly stave off osteoporosis in your future (if you don't get enough calcium, your body will dip into its own supply to make breastmilk). This doesn't mean, however, that you should drink a gallon of cow's milk every day. In fact, too much milk ingested by a new mother may upset a nursing baby's stomach, and it doesn't take milk to make milk. If you enjoy drinking cow's milk, by all means, have two to four glasses per day. There are other good sources of calcium, however, including yogurt, cheese, cottage cheese, broccoli, leafy greens, tofu prepared with calcium, calcium-fortified orange juice, salmon, sesame seeds, corn tortillas, and blackstrap molasses.

As often as possible, try to eat foods with multiple nutrients. Broccoli, for example, is a fantastic choice, supplying high levels of calcium, plus vitamin C and other antioxidants. Dairy products have calcium and protein. Dried apricots have beta carotene and iron. Dried legumes have iron and protein. In general, you will probably find that monitoring every bite takes too much of your time and you won't keep it up. Instead, eat a wide variety of foods and make sure almost everything you eat is densely nutritious. Avoiding a nutritional rut will ensure that you're taking in a good selection of nutrients, so experiment with different types of grains, cheeses, fruits, and vegetables. Be a culinary adventurer; your body (and your baby!) will thank you. And don't forget to drink a lot of water and juice. Juice diluted with spring

Take a Cue from Your Nursing Baby

You would do well to imitate your nursing baby's relaxed concentration at mealtime. Feeding is her great happiness and is very serious business indeed—requiring her full powers of attention and producing profound satisfaction. Find the lesson in her joy of feeding! Remember that eating is a life-affirming and -sustaining activity. Just as she's learning her first life-lessons from her experience of breastfeeding, you can reconnect to the importance and joy of eating by watching your little one and returning to an appreciation of one of the fundamental truths of living!

Practice mindful eating. Choose healthy foods that fuel your body for optimal health and provide your baby with the best nutrients through your breastmilk. After all, you wouldn't expect your car to run well if you started putting the wrong fuel in it! Also, concentrate fully on the act of eating while you are doing it. Chew every bite and really taste your food. Appreciate the nourishment you give to your body. In other words, pay attention to what you are eating, why you are eating it, and how you are eating it. You may be surprised at what you find. Your baby has the right idea.

water or seltzer water is a healthy but less caloric choice than straight juice. Fresh fruit and vegetable juices are wonderful, and a good juicer is a healthy investment if you use it regularly.

Move Over, Meat: Other Sources of Protein

Meat, poultry, even seafood, although packed with protein and other nutrients, are also packed with cholesterol and, especially

OMEGA-3 FATTY ACID: DHA

Nutritionists at the Institute of Food Technologists in Chicago have recently released findings that a substance called DHA, omega-3 fatty acid, may be important to the development of a newborn's brain. DHA is found naturally in breastmilk, but it is not in infant formula. Consuming two servings of fish or shellfish per week before and after giving birth can boost DHA levels in breastmilk. Fish high in DHA include salmon, sardines, and mackerel.

the way they are produced these days, filled with hormones, antibiotics, and in the case of fish, industrial toxins from polluted waters. Consumed in smaller amounts, however, meat and fish can be nutritional allies. If you eat meat, try to find organic, free-range meat. Make sure fish is fresh and purchase it only from reputable grocers.

Use meats and fish as means of flavoring your food, not as main ingredients. Instead, feature dishes based on grains—such as pasta, brown rice, kasha (buckwheat groats), and polenta—or serve vegetable entrees. Flavor your stir-fry with a few small pieces of minced chicken or fish, add just a half cup or so of lean ground beef to a batch of spaghetti sauce, or mince just a few shrimp and stir into a big batch of yellow rice and vegetables for a lighter interpretation of jambalaya. And don't forget soy! Recent studies show that adding soy to your diet can significantly reduce cholesterol, protecting you against the risk of heart disease—and soy also has anticancer properties that may add protection against breast cancer. Soybeans are an excellent source of protein and versatile, widely available now in many forms, such as soy flour (replace two or three tablespoons of white flour with soy flour in baking), tofu (kids love it—it's mild, cheeselike, and

POPULAR DIETS AND BREASTFEEDING

Before embarking on any postdelivery diet strategy, be sure to consult your doctor. Any weight-loss regimen or drastic change in the nutritional content of your diet should be discussed with your health care team; you want the best diet to ensure your health—and your baby's. Here are some of the diet choices that run the gamut of personal, lifestyle, and nutritional preferences.

Pritikin Diet. A low-fat, -cholesterol, -protein, and -refined-carbohydrate diet emphasizing whole, unrefined, minimally processed carbohydrates such as grains, fruits, and vegetables. Although not vegetarian, animal products are consumed only in small amounts. The diet was developed with the express purpose of reversing coronary heart disease, but is a good idea for everyone! The complete Pritikin Program also includes aerobic exercise.

Macrobiotics. A holistic, individualized way of living in harmony with your surroundings, which includes a whole-grain-centered diet and food that is locally available and in season (rather than shipped from other locations). Use of animal products is limited but not eliminated. This diet is generally very healthy, although some foods common to macrobiotic diets, such as miso (a fermented soy soup base), are quite salty. Look for macrobiotic cooking classes in your area or books on how to follow the diet.

Lacto-ovo-vegetarianism. Vegetarians follow the practice of avoiding meat, fowl, and sometimes fish, for moral or nutritional reasons. A lacto-ovo-vegetarian diet—a good choice for nursing mothers—includes foods of plant origin, such as vegetables, fruits, grains, beans, and nuts, and dairy products, such as milk, cream, butter, yogurt, cheese, and eggs. The diet achieves maximum benefit when only nonfat or low-fat dairy products are consumed. See page 114 for special diet tips for vegetarian mothers.

McDougall Diet. This vegan vegetarian diet (absolutely no animal products, only plant-based foods) is cholesterol-free, low in fat, sugar, and salt, and high in complex carbohydrates and fiber. The diet is healthy, but those accustomed to a standard American diet may find it difficult to stick to. It can, however, have dramatic health benefits, although breastfeeding mothers must be careful to get adequate nutrients on a vegan diet (see page 114).

great when cubed and marinated for stir-fry), soy milk (perfect with cereal), texturized vegetable protein (TVP; a great ground meat substitute), or even soybeans themselves, roasted in the oven for a delicious, crunchy snack.

Vitamins and Supplements

The debate about the efficacy of nutritional supplements rages on, and although some say taking vitamins and minerals is a waste of money, there is compelling evidence that some supplements can make a difference. If you always eat a perfectly balanced variety of healthy, organically grown food produced in nutrient-rich soil, then you can probably forgo the supplements. Most of us, however, despite our best efforts, often find ourselves at the end of the day short of necessary nutrients. A multivitamin and mineral supplement or prenatal supplement with levels at or slightly above the Recommended Daily Allowance (RDA) is a good insurance policy. (Make sure any vitamin or supplement you buy includes a notice that it has been routinely dissolution tested and approved per the official U.S. Pharmacopeia (USP) Standards.)

The nursing mother, however, has to be particularly careful about taking supplements. Avoid supplements that offer so-called megadoses. Too much of certain vitamins and minerals can be harmful to you, and even at levels your adult system can handle, they might be toxic to your baby. Iron is a perfect example. Nursing mothers who take iron supplements may be harming their babies by giving them more iron than their tiny bodies can handle. Many supplements that are healthy additions to the diet of an adult should be avoided when nursing. For example, high doses of vitamins C, E, and A, in the form of beta carotene, an antioxidant, have been shown to have cancer-fighting properties. Garlic supplements have antibiotic effects, ginseng is purported to increase energy, and gingko to boost memory. All these supplements are great choices for a new father's diet, but until you are finished nursing, do not take any supplements beyond your prenatal vitamin, unless your doctor has advised you otherwise. (Feel free to add fresh garlic and natural sources of vitamin C to your diet, however. You won't be receiving the megadoses you'd get in supplements this way, but you'll still reap the benefits. Note that vitamin C levels must be replenished in the body each day for maximum healthy effect. Have a glass of fresh orange juice every morning and fresh produce throughout the day.)

If you know you aren't getting enough calcium in your diet, ask your doctor about supplementing it with calcium citrate; calcium in this form is the most easily absorbed by the body. You may also want to ask about supplementing your diet with spirulina, an alga high in protein, calcium, and vitamin B_{12}. An extremely nutritious food, spirulina can be purchased in the supplement section of your local natural or health food store. If you buy it in powder form, you may have to get used to the taste.

Folic acid is also required in increased quantities by nursing mothers. Natural foods high in folic acid include raspberries, oranges, pineapple, asparagus, spinach, lentils, wheat germ, peanuts, and chicken livers. However, there is some evidence that fortified foods, such as vitamin-fortified bran cereals, and supplements provide a better pathway for the absorption of folic acid in the body, which can be destroyed through cooking. Some tips to preserve the folic acid content of foods: Cut food into large chunks before cooking, not small pieces. Using only a small amount of water, steam or simmer foods, and avoid overcooking. Eat as many raw fruits and vegetables as you can. As of January 1998, all manufacturers must add folic acid to enriched products. Folic acid is a B vitamin, and not getting the right amount in the early days of pregnancy increases the risk of some birth defects. According to the National Academy of Sciences, women of childbearing age should consume 400 micrograms of folic acid daily, but most only take in about 200 micrograms. Folic acid is also being shown to help prevent heart disease and may help reduce the risk of some cancers. Nursing mothers should be sure to get this important vitamin into their daily diets.

Unless prescribed by your physician, never feed your baby any kind of vitamin or supplement. Your little one should be receiving all her nutrients from your breastmilk. If something more than your milk is needed, your doctor will advise you.

Eat Whole Foods

Choose fresh produce over frozen, frozen over canned. Buy whole oats instead of instant oatmeal, brown rice instead of white, whole wheat products instead of those made with white flour. Whenever possible, choose the least processed food available. Whole foods are closer to their natural form and therefore retain more nutrients and require fewer chemicals to preserve, flavor, and color them. Avoid foods with a lot of chemical additives. Additives may keep old food from spoiling, but who wants to eat old food? When the season is right, check out your local farmers' market or produce stands, both great sources of fresh, whole food.

ORGANICS: WORTH THE PRICE?

Many supermarkets now carry at least a small selection of organic produce, flours, grains, beans, pastas, and other organic foods. You may be reluctant to try organics because they cost more. Why spend $3.50 for a package of organic whole wheat spaghetti when you can get the same amount of regular spaghetti for $1.50? According to California Certified Organic Farmers (CCOF), organic food costs more because organic production costs and risks are higher, environmentally friendly farming practices cost more, and state registration and certification costs add to the price (there is currently no federal organic certification process). Yet, if you consider the health and environmental costs and risks of eating food treated with pesticides, chemical fertilizers, waxes, dyes, and preservatives, the relative price of buying organic food seems less extreme. Buying and eating organic is an investment in your family's health as well as the earth's health. Organic food has other advantages, too:

◎ *Without preservatives, organic food won't last as long, so it will be shipped to you sooner and you will be eating fresher food (who knows how long that bright, shiny apple beneath a thick coat of wax has been carted around the country?).*

◎ *Organic food is generally far less processed and contains more of the whole food, retaining more nutrients (for example, the whole wheat versus the regular spaghetti).*

◎ *Organic food tastes better. An organic, vine-ripened, fresh-picked tomato bears little resemblance to the bland, pink, grainy "vegetables" on sale at your local supermarket.*

◎ *Organic milk doesn't contain bovine growth hormones. Choose meat and eggs from free-range chickens; these animals are not fed or treated with hormones or antibiotics. The hormones may increase your risk of breast cancer and other diseases, and are being closely studied now.*

◎ *Organic food doesn't promote the pollution of the planet.*

Note: Because organics aren't federally regulated, verifying that food is truly organic may take a little detective work. Ask your grocer about the organic food in your local store. Can you see proof that the grower is certified (a process in some states requiring inspections)? Was the food grown nearby, or shipped from another state? If your grocer doesn't know, find another grocer. Farmers' markets, health and natural food stores, and roadside produce stands are often good sources for organic produce grown in your region. Also, there are many good direct mail suppliers of organic foods (see Appendix B, "Resources," on page 271).

At the very least, if you cannot find organic food, wash your produce! Avoid buying fruits and vegetables coated in wax, which is an efficient pesticide trap (common with apples and cucumbers, for example), or dyed (common in oranges—check the label). Again, ask your grocer, if produce isn't labeled but looks waxy or artificially bright.

When you get your produce home, soak it in a sink full of water with a splash of vinegar, or scrub it with lots of dish soap and a vegetable brush or scouring pad reserved for this purpose. If you do end up with waxed or dyed skin on your produce, peel the fruit or veggie—but remember that nutrients are concentrated in the skins of many fruits and vegetables, so organic or thoroughly washed produce is a better choice.

SPECIAL TIPS FOR VEGETARIAN MOTHERS

◎ Be creative in getting the extra protein you need, especially if you are a vegan vegetarian and don't eat dairy products at all. Eat plenty of legumes, grains, soy products (soy flour, soy milk, tofu, texturized vegetable protein, and soybeans), seeds, nuts, and nut butters. If you do eat dairy, low-or nonfat milk, yogurt, and cheese, as well as eggs, are all good protein sources.

◎ Get your calcium! If you are a vegan, be sure to eat lots of broccoli, collard greens, kale, or other leafy greens. Sea vegetables are excellent sources of both calcium and protein (check your Asian grocery or natural food store). Calcium-fortified orange juice, soy milk, and tofu are great choices. Blackstrap molasses contains calcium and iron, too.

◎ Add wheat germ. Stir wheat germ into brown rice, oatmeal, grits, bread dough, and batters for an extra nutritional punch.

◎ Although some sources say otherwise, vitamin B_{12} can be found solely in animal products, including dairy products. Talk to your doctor about taking a B_{12} supplement. This vitamin is also found in spirulina, an alga.

◎ If you are a vegan and live in an area where there are more clouds than sun, you might need to add vitamin D to your diet. Talk to your doctor.

◎ You don't eat meat, so you'll need more iron. Dried fruit, legumes, soybeans and tofu, spinach, and blackstrap molasses are all iron-rich.

WHAT A NURSING MOM SHOULD *NOT* EAT

Just as important as eating the right things is not eating the wrong things. These offenders fall into two categories, neither of which, perhaps surprisingly, has anything to do with upsetting a baby's stomach. Although some people claim that certain foods that cause an adult digestive problems will cause the same in a breast-feeding baby, many mothers swear this isn't true. As far as garlic, spices, broccoli, beans, and other such gas-producing foods are concerned, if you like them, eat them. If your baby becomes suddenly upset or flatulent, maybe they are causing a problem. Experiment. More important are the two more insidious offenders: mood-altering substances (caffeine, alcohol, nicotine, and other drugs), which are bad for your baby, and the often craved yet insidious combination of sugar and fat, which is bad for you.

CAFFEINE: YOUR BABY TAKES MILK WITH HIS COFFEE?

According to most sources, one or two cups of coffee per day won't affect your baby. On the other hand, his system isn't able to eliminate caffeine as fast as yours can, so the caffeine he gets from you can accumulate in his body. If you've abstained from your morning coffee all through pregnancy and are dying to resume the habit, you

BECOME *A*WARE OF EVERYTHING *Y*OU *E*AT

Before you take a bite, ask yourself: "Would I give this to my baby?" If not, think twice. What could you eat instead?

might want to consider giving it up for good. Caffeine has absolutely no nutritional value and if you've been off it for nine months, you've broken any physical addiction. Why start up again?

If you are very attached to a cozy cup of morning coffee and you just can't stand herbal tea (a good substitute for those who enjoy it), you know that if you drink one cup it won't quickly lead to drinking six cups, and, after a week or two of trying it, you don't notice any ill effects in your baby such as excessive wakefulness, go ahead and indulge. Or try decaffeinated coffee

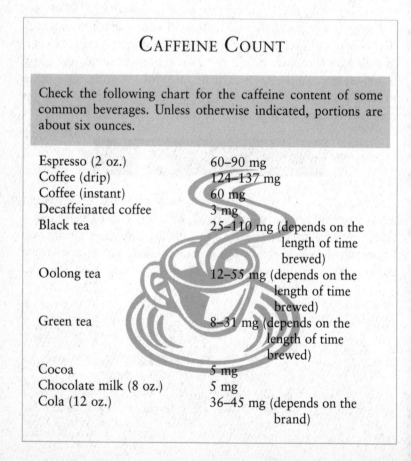

CAFFEINE COUNT

Check the following chart for the caffeine content of some common beverages. Unless otherwise indicated, portions are about six ounces.

Espresso (2 oz.)	60–90 mg
Coffee (drip)	124–137 mg
Coffee (instant)	60 mg
Decaffeinated coffee	3 mg
Black tea	25–110 mg (depends on the length of time brewed)
Oolong tea	12–55 mg (depends on the length of time brewed)
Green tea	8–31 mg (depends on the length of time brewed)
Cocoa	5 mg
Chocolate milk (8 oz.)	5 mg
Cola (12 oz.)	36–45 mg (depends on the brand)

HERBS AND HERBAL REMEDIES

Many herbal preparations, including teas, infusions, tinctures, and tablets, are touted as healthful treatments for a variety of ills. Herbs can be wonderful healers, but for the breastfeeding mother, they can also be dangerous. Many powerful prescription drugs are made from herbs, and when used incorrectly or without sufficient guidance or knowledge, herbal remedies can be dangerous, especially for your baby. A dosage that helps you may be harmful to an infant. Therefore, unless an herb has been specifically prescribed to you by a physician or reputable and responsible herbalist who knows you are breastfeeding, avoid taking herbs, including medicinal herbal teas.

However, the types of herbs and spices used in cooking are good for teas and broths and for adding flavor to your meals (herbs are the leaves of fragrant plants, whereas spices are made from the seeds, roots, bark, and stems of plants and trees). Ginger, peppermint, cinnamon, spearmint, apple, orange, lemon, or other fruit teas are all fine. Just be sure your choice of tea doesn't contain actual tea leaves. Chamomile tea can also be soothing. However, if you are allergic to ragweed, avoid chamomile, as it is in the ragweed family and could produce an allergic reaction. For other soothing, warm drinks, warm a mug of juice and flavor it with a dash of cinnamon, or savor a hot cup of lemon water (spring water with a squeeze of fresh lemon), which is a great system cleanser. Or try a broth made by boiling a clove of garlic and half a small onion (garlic has great antibacterial effects, opens lungs and bronchial tubes, and may even help to inhibit tumor cell formation).

The following cooking herbs and spices are fine in moderation, and make a good base for any cook. If you would like to try others, ask your doctor or trained herbalist about the safety of particular herbs for nursing mothers.

SAFE HERBS

Basil	Oregano
Bay leaf	Parsley
Dill	Rosemary
Mint (great for tea—a good digestive aid after a meal)	Sage
	Tarragon
	Thyme

SAFE SPICES

Black pepper	Ginger (great in tea for colds, colitis, and nausea, plus it aids digestion and circulation)
Cayenne pepper (great for clogged sinuses)	
Cinnamon (great for tea)	
Cloves (great for tea)	Nutmeg
Cumin	Paprika

Aromatherapy, the therapeutic use of essential oils of flowers, leaves, roots, or other parts of plants by inhalation or absorption through the skin, may be relaxing and beneficial—physiologically and psychologically—to new mothers. Eucalyptus oil in a new mother's bathwater is invigorating, for example, and orange oil is relaxing. However, essential oils can be extremely toxic, even lethal, to infants. Keep oils safely out of the reach of infants and small children and handle them with the same care and respect you give to handling medications, or forgo the use of essential oils in the house until children are older.

(choose the type decaffeinated with water instead of chemicals). Decaf still has a small amount of caffeine, however, so don't overdo it. Postum or other grain-based "coffees" are completely caffeine-free and if you get used to them, they can be a more-than-adequate substitute for that beloved cup of Joe.

If your passion is cola or hot tea or some other source of caffeine, the same applies. A little is probably just fine. A lot is bad for you and may begin to affect your baby. If you crave carbonation, try seltzer (club soda without the salt), or ginger ale (again, in moderation—ginger ale has a lot of sugar). Avoid diet sodas because the effects of aspartame have yet to be seen, and many claim it causes headaches in adults and seizures in children. If you are a die-hard tea drinker, try switching from black tea to Chinese varieties, such as Oolong or green tea, both of which have less caffeine. Green tea has been in the news a lot lately as a potential cancer fighter. The health benefits of an occasional cup of green tea may far outweigh the relatively small amount of caffeine you'll ingest.

ALCOHOL: BOTTLES UP!

The thought of giving your baby alcohol is probably shocking, yet many breastfeeding mothers will have an occasional alcoholic beverage, especially after the first few months. Like caffeine, small amounts of alcohol (one glass of wine or beer) probably won't harm your baby, though he will probably feel the effects somewhat. If you want to have a drink, wait until the last feeding for the night, and then limit yourself to one or two. By morning, the effects of the alcohol in your milk will be minimal, unless, of course, you have overindulged. If you drink too much, not only will your baby drink too much, but you will be less alert and able to handle any emergencies that might arise. Drinking and motherhood don't mix. You'll also want to be careful about foods that contain alcohol, such as entrees with wine sauces or desserts soaked in brandy. Avoid liquors and mixed drinks altogether.

If you're drawn to an occasional glass of beer or wine as a way to relax when you sit down in your nursing haven to breastfeed your baby, consider this: A study by scientists at the Monell Chemical Sense Center in Philadelphia showed that when mothers drank orange juice mixed with the amount of alcohol commonly contained in a can of beer, their babies drank an average of 22 percent less milk than when the same mothers drank an equivalent amount of pure juice at another nursing session. If you are looking for ways to relax and enjoy feeding times, check out chapter 7 for some wonderful tips on relaxation and stress-management that are better for you—and for your baby—than alcohol.

Also, although results vary in a number of studies that have been done on the effects of alcohol on breast cancer risk, most health practitioners agree that even moderate alcohol consumption (three or four drinks per week) may increase your risk of premenopausal breast cancer an average of 30 percent. Yes, *thirty percent!*

NICOTINE

Nicotine is more dangerous for the fetus than for the nursing baby. We hope that if you smoke, you managed to quit while pregnant. If you didn't, there are still reasons to quit now. Nicotine is perhaps the most difficult addiction to break. You may need help. Talk to your doctor for recommendations.

Heavy smoking (over a pack a day) has been shown to decrease a mother's milk supply and, in rare cases, cause nausea, vomiting, abdominal pain, and diarrhea in the nursing baby. Smoking less than a pack a day probably won't affect your baby adversely, as far as nicotine is concerned (it will go into his system, but will be metabolized fairly quickly). However, secondhand smoke is a serious health hazard. According to the National Institutes of Health and the National Cancer Institute, secondhand smoke is associated with as many as three hundred thousand cases of bronchitis and pneumonia each year in infants and children up to eighteen months of age. Secondhand smoke also increases the chances for middle ear problems, causes coughing and wheezing, and worsens asthma conditions. Even more compelling is the evidence that parental smoking may increase an infant's chances of dying from sudden infant death syndrome,

FATHER ALERT!

YOU'RE NOT NURSING— WHY SHOULD YOU QUIT?

Too much alcohol, coffee, nicotine, or overuse of medication and other drugs is unhealthy, but you are only hurting yourself, right? Well . . . although it is true that your baby isn't receiving unhealthy substances directly through you, there are several compelling reasons for you to kick the habit, too. For one thing, your partner will find it much easier to forgo that morning cup of coffee or evening cocktail if you aren't indulging in front of her. For another, your child is watching you and before you know it, he'll be trying to do everything you do. Also, breaking bad habits will make you healthier and might increase your lifespan.

especially when the baby sleeps with one or more smoking parents. Is smoking worth all that? In addition, cigarettes and matches pose a serious choking hazard to your baby, and matches and lighters could spell disaster with young children who figure out how to make fire.

If you absolutely can't quit or won't quit (as we said, it is a powerful addiction), at the very least avoid smoking around your child (including when you are together in the car) and preferably never smoke in the house. Children whose parents smoke have a higher chance of becoming smokers themselves. On top of risks to your child, smoking increases your chances of lung and cervical cancer, among other health problems. Many, many smokers have quit successfully and are enjoying the health benefits. You can be one of them!

MEDICATIONS AND OTHER DRUGS

The American Academy of Pediatrics (AAP) has developed three risk categories concerning drugs during breastfeeding: (1) drugs that should not be taken while breastfeeding, (2) drugs that require temporary interruption of breastfeeding, and (3) drugs that are compatible with breastfeeding. Always tell your doctor and your pharmacist you are breastfeeding, and talk to your health care providers to determine whether any prescription or over-the-counter drug recommended for you—from a simple antacid or analgesic to an antidepressant, barbiturate, or specific antibiotic—is safe for your nursing baby.

The long-term effects to an infant from ingesting the breast-milk of mothers who take birth control pills while breastfeeding hasn't been determined. Some experts believe that the progestin-only minipill is safe if nursing mothers wait about four to six weeks, until the breastfeeding relationship is well under way; this pill, however, can cause spotting and is a less effective contraceptive than the estrogen-progestin combinations, which can decrease milk supply. It may be prudent to avoid oral contraceptives and use another form of contraception when breastfeeding, such as a diaphragm or condom used in combination with a spermicide.

In the January 1994 issue of *Pediatrics,* the American Academy of Pediatrics included the following in a list of medications that are usually compatible with breastfeeding:

◎ *acetaminophen*

◎ *many antibiotics*

◎ *antiepileptics (although Primidone should be given with caution)*

◎ *most antihistamines*

◎ *most antihypertensives*

- *aspirin (should be used with caution—acetaminophen is a preferable option)*

- *caffeine (moderate amounts in drinks or food only—never caffeine pills!)*

- *codeine*

- *decongestants*

- *ibuprofen*

- *insulin*

- *quinine*

- *thyroid medications*

According to the Food and Drug Administration (FDA), the following drugs are definitely *not* safe while nursing. Avoid:

- *Radioactive drugs used for some diagnostic tests, like gallium-69, iodine-125, iodine-131, or technetium-99m (these can be taken while breastfeeding if you stop nursing temporarily—continue to pump and discard your breastmilk, and feed the baby breastmilk frozen ahead of time or formula until the drugs are out of your system).*

- *Bromocriptine (Parlodel): A drug for Parkinson's disease, it will also decrease your milk supply.*

- *Most chemotherapy drugs for cancer: Since they kill cells in your body, they may harm the baby as well.*

- *Ergotamine (for migraine headaches): Causes vomiting, diarrhea, and convulsions in infants.*

- *Lithium (for manic-depressive illness): Excreted in human milk.*

- *Methotrexate (for arthritis): Can suppress the baby's immune system.*

⊚ *Drugs of abuse: Some drugs, such as cocaine and PCP, can intoxicate the baby. Others, such as amphetamines, heroin, and marijuana, can cause irritability, poor sleeping patterns, tremors, and vomiting. Babies become addicted to these drugs.*

⊚ *Tobacco smoke and nicotine (see page 120).*

SUGAR AND FAT: THE DIABOLICAL DUO

Have you ever noticed that if you start the morning with doughnuts or, worse yet, a candy bar, you crave sugar all day long? Take a second look at what the Food Pyramid for Nursing Mothers recommends about fat and sugar: *Use sparingly.* The following are some great reasons to try to avoid this health-destroying combination:

1. Sugar and fat fill you up during a meal so you don't have room for more healthy, nutrient-dense foods.

HOMEOPATHIC REMEDIES

Homeopathy is a therapy based on the principle that if a particular remedy produces symptoms in a healthy person, that same remedy will cure a sick person displaying those same symptoms. Remedies consist of extremely small doses of herbs and other substances, diluted and shaken. Many homeopathic remedies are available over the counter and are generally considered safer than prescription drugs, but exercise caution when breastfeeding and don't take anything not prescribed by a licensed naturopathic physician, your M.D., your OB/GYN, or your pediatrician.

2. Sugar and fat increase your appetite for more sugar and fat, and decrease your appetite for healthy food. The more you eat, the more extreme the effect.

3. Sugar-fat foods are commonly loaded with preservatives and chemicals.

4. Sugar-fat foods are usually low in fiber and can promote irregularity.

5. Sugar-fat foods promote tooth decay.

6. Sugar-fat foods cause extreme rises and drops in blood sugar, resulting in a feeling of dragginess and fatigue that is difficult to overcome except by consuming more sugar-fat foods.

7. Sugar-fat foods can contribute to the development of diabetes and obesity and have been linked to increased risk of breast and colon cancer, as well as heart disease—definitely not good news!

8. Sugar is not needed in your diet in any amount. Fat is only needed in small amounts.

Also, beware of food labels that proclaim a product to be "nonfat" or "fat free." Many nonfat foods are loaded with sugar, and because sugar converts to fat in the body, an entire box of nonfat cookies can still go straight to your thighs! In addition to reading the fat content—or even the calorie content—of foods, look at the list of ingredients. Better yet, bake your own; a home-made batch of oatmeal cookies made with organic oats, honey, wheat germ, raisins, and applesauce is a far superior choice of dessert than a box of processed, nonfat cookies.

If you try to cut sugar from your diet, you will probably notice intense cravings for it, especially in the first few weeks. If you can last through this period, sweets will seem far less appealing and you will be able to tolerate less sugar when you do indulge. How do you get through the first few weeks? It isn't easy. One of the best things you can do is to eliminate all sources of sweets from your home. In addition, keep a lot of healthy snack foods handy. Sugar-fat foods are easy to grab and eat quickly. Remove this temptation. You and your baby will receive far more nutrients and reap the healthy benefits of eating foods that have true nutritional value. Sugar doesn't!

A 1994 health survey indicated that 70 percent of people queried believed they had healthy diet habits—yet the diets they described were way too high in fat, with not enough fresh vegetables and fruits or carbohydrates (from the Food Pyramid's grain group). Don't fall into this trap. Ideally, you should strive for a diet that includes only 20 to 30 percent of calories from fat (and that means choosing low- or nonfat foods that are sugar-free!).

One graphic but surefire way to tell if you are consuming too many sugar-fat foods: examine your stool after using the bathroom. If it is hard, composed of compacted marblelike balls, and floats, you are eating too much fat and sugar and not enough fiber. If it is smooth, excreted in one long column, and sinks, your diet is lower in fat and contains a good amount of fiber.

Making healthy diet choices is well worth the effort. And the transition from breastmilk to pure, healthy, whole foods will be an easy and natural one for your child if the rest of the family already eats in this holistic manner. According to the September 1997 issue of *Pediatrics,* young people between the ages of two and nineteen receive 40 percent of their energy from fat and added sugar and only 1 percent of children and teenagers eat truly healthy diets. A USDA telephone survey revealed that the diets of 16 percent of 3,307 young people interviewed did not meet *any* of the federal guidelines for nutrition. A nutritionist at Stanford University Medical Center asserts, "It is in early childhood when you have the groundwork

Delicious, Healthy, Quick Snacks

◎ Fresh fruit, such as apples, bananas, peaches, pears, and grapes

◎ Dried fruit (very sweet), such as raisins, dried apricots, and prunes

◎ Washed and cut-up raw vegetables, such as carrots, celery, radishes, pea pods, broccoli, and cauliflower

◎ Frozen produce. Pop it like candy! Try peas, carrots, and green beans. You can also freeze green grapes on a cookie sheet then store in a freezer bag. These are absolutely delicious. Try freezing other fruit, too, such as strawberries, sliced peaches, and bananas.

◎ Whole-grain crackers (read the label—many contain sugar)

◎ Popcorn (low-fat microwave varieties are fast and easy, but plain old buttered popcorn can be surprisingly caloric—remember, it's what you put on it that turns any kind of popcorn into an undesirable high-fat snack!)

◎ Pretzels (low- or no-salt are best)

as to what foods will become favorite foods. Parents need to set an example and remember they are in charge of the food purchased." Let your goal be to make all your baby's meals just as healthy as his nursing meals have been. You and your spouse or partner will benefit from eating right, too. Healthy eating is a family affair!

CALCULATING THE FAT CONTENT OF FOODS FROM FOOD LABELS

Keep in mind that the percentage of fat listed on food labels often shows the percentage calculated by *weight,* not by calories. To figure out the percentage of calories from fat per serving for any food, you'll need to do this simple math. Multiply the number of grams of fat in a serving by 9 (each gram of fat produces 9 calories), divide this by the total number of calories per serving, and multiply by 100. If the percentage of calories from fat is more than 30 percent, you're looking at a high-fat item!

For example, consider the fat content of a cinnamon roll: One serving contains 250 calories and weighs 56 grams. The fat content is 13 grams and the total percentage of fat by weight is 19 percent. But, let's do the calculation: 13 grams of fat × 9 = 117; 117 ÷ 250 calories per serving = .468; .468 × 100 = 46.8. That's 46.8 percent of calories from fat per serving! Lots of fat but not much nutritive value for you or your baby.

A BABY AT THE TABLE

Even when your child is still very young, she can participate in family meals. She can join you on the table in her infant seat the day you bring her home from the hospital, if she isn't crying, and as soon as she is old enough to sit in a high chair, she can participate even more. (The age babies are high-chair ready varies widely, but when your baby can sit up without slumping over and can hold her head up well, you can try the high chair. Be sure she's belted in!) Babies are social and love to see what you are doing. Putting her in view of the table, even in her nearby infant swing, and including her in your conversations can be fun for the whole family. If your infant starts to scream, however, a pleasant family meal can be transformed into a nightmare of indigestion, so if she doesn't do well at the table or is hungry or tired, tend to her needs, then have your dinner later. Before long, she'll be a natural part of the family meals.

Even when your baby is old enough to start eating solids, you may want to feed her first and feed yourself after she has gone to bed. (That doesn't mean she can't sit with you when you eat earlier meals, even if her actual meal is at a different time.) Some parents enjoy eating and feeding their baby at the same time. It depends on your family and how you like your meals. Do what works for you.

After four to six months of exclusive breastfeeding, you are probably looking forward to your little one's first taste of solids. That thin rice cereal may not look like much, but to your baby, it is a major leap forward; for you, too, it signals the first step in a

DON'T RUSH IT

As eager as you may be to begin feeding your baby solids, remember that he doesn't need anything other than breast-milk for six months. If he is eager to try other foods at four months, by all means, indulge him. If he isn't ready, how-ever, don't push it. If he cries, spits out all the food, pushes out every bite with his tongue, or doesn't seem to enjoy the experience, put away the tiny spoon for another few weeks. You will get mighty tired of shoveling those inefficiently small spoonfuls of food into that bottomless pit far sooner than you can imagine, and you always want to keep eating experiences positive for your child.

FEEDING TIP

When you first begin to feed your baby solid foods, it can be helpful to offer the breast first, to take the edge off his hunger. A hungry baby can become frustrated when he isn't able to get enough solids down to satisfy, leading to a miserable feeding experience for everyone involved. A less hungry baby may be in a better state of mind for experimenting.

On the other hand, some babies, when offered the breast first, quickly become full and aren't interested in eating any solids at all. If this is the case, he may not be ready to start solids yet. Or try offering solids before the breast, when he may be more eager, then finishing off with a breastfeeding to be sure he has enough food in his tummy.

In other words, see what works for your baby.

long and complex weaning process. Don't worry, she won't be off the breast for quite a while yet (unless you wean her on purpose). After six months, however, breastmilk alone is no longer enough. Your baby will need the additional nutrition solid foods provide, so this is the time to introduce her to the wonderful world of solids.

Much as you may long to develop your child's palate into that of the sophisticated gourmet, be aware that her digestive system is inexperienced. Foods must be introduced gradually, allowing her to adjust. Complex proteins, such as those in dairy products, egg whites, and meats, should be introduced carefully and one at a time, because these substances can produce allergic reactions in babies whose systems aren't yet sufficiently mature to handle them.

Start with a single-grain cereal such as rice or oatmeal, thinned with breastmilk. You can make these yourself, or buy the boxed cereal (more nutritious than the jars because contain added iron). Try to find the organic, whole grain varieties. Single-ingredient yellow vegetables (carrots, butternut squash) can be sampled next. Introducing vegetables before fruits helps to avoid a baby refusing all solid food but that which is sweet. After you have tried a few vegetables, you can introduce fruits, such as peaches, pears, and apples. Pureed meat, such as chicken or turkey, can be introduced at six to eight months if you plan to feed meat to your baby, as can plain yogurt, with your doctor's approval. Most doctors recommend waiting to introduce whole milk and egg whites until the end of the first year. Shellfish and all nut products should wait until the end of the second year, as these are common allergens.

SIGNS YOUR BABY IS READY FOR SOLIDS

- ◎ He shows interest in your food or in the eating process.

- ◎ She suddenly seems hungry all the time, even though she is getting plenty of breastmilk.

- ◎ When given a small spoonful of cereal, he swallows it rather than pushing it all back out with his tongue (all babies push out food at first because the tongue must thrust forward during nursing, but babies ready for solids will soon figure out that a different process is required for swallowing solid food).

- ◎ She is able to hold her head up quite well. A baby must have firm control over her head before she can be expected to master a new swallowing technique.

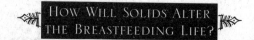

BEST FOODS FOR A BABY'S FIRST YEAR

The following chart shows which foods you can introduce to your baby as he matures. Introduce new foods one at a time, waiting several days before trying something new. Signs of allergy include swelling around the mouth and face, wheezing, skin rashes, stomach cramps, and diarrhea. Food allergies are not as common as some would have you believe, but they can be serious so caution is advised. Also, allergies are often outgrown, so a baby allergic to wheat or milk may not always be so. Call your doctor if you suspect your baby is having an allergic reaction to any food.

HOW WILL SOLIDS ALTER THE BREASTFEEDING LIFE?

You may be wondering what will be different about breastfeeding a baby who also eats solid foods. Not much, except that the baby probably won't breastfeed quite as often. On the other hand, the baby may breastfeed just as often, especially at first, when she isn't actually getting much food into her stomach (sometimes you'll wonder if anything at all ended up in there!).

When your baby's intake of breastmilk decreases, you may notice a corresponding decrease in your milk supply. As long as you keep breastfeeding regularly, however, you will produce as much milk as your baby needs. You may also experience the return of your menstrual period. On the other hand, it may not return until months after you have weaned your baby completely. Every woman's body is different.

Emotionally, you may begin to feel the first pangs of separation. Your baby is eating regular food. How long will it be until she doesn't need you at all? Rest assured, it will be a very, very long time. Sustaining the breastfeeding relationship for at least a year (the minimum length of time recommended by the American Academy of Pediatrics) can help to maintain your physical and emotional

BABY'S AGE	FOODS TO TRY
At four to six months Foods in this category are your baby's first foods, and should be pure, smooth, and absolutely without added salt, sugar, modified food starch, or other additives. Thinning any food with breastmilk is acceptable. However, if you have added breastmilk to any food, throw away all unused portions; don't save them for the next meal. Also, if you have dipped a used spoon into any baby food, throw away unused portions. Bacteria can grow quickly in baby food, and your baby's delicate system isn't yet as hardy as yours. Better safe than sorry!	dry cereals (thin with breastmilk): brown rice, oatmeal, barley mashed ripe banana strained applesauce cooked and pureed vegetables: carrots, butternut squash, green beans, peas, sweet potatoes cooked and pureed fruits: pears, apricots, peaches, prunes, plums, nectarines plain yogurt (O.K. this with your doctor)
At six to eight months This is the age to experiment with a wider range of foods. Don't expect your baby to like everything, but don't expect her to dislike foods you dislike, either. Try not to show any bias. She will hardly want to eat a spoonful of plain yogurt if you offer it while making a horrible face and saying "yucky!" Be pleasant and	other cereals: Cream of Wheat, wheat germ (good for stirring into oatmeal), slightly thicker oatmeal and rice cereals other vegetables, cooked and pureed or mashed: asparagus, yellow squash, corn, potatoes, broccoli, spinach, beets, root vegetables (turnips, rutabagas, parsnips), okra

BABY'S AGE	FOODS TO TRY
mildly excited about each new offering, and explore her culinary tastes. Remember, just because she spits something out the first time doesn't mean she doesn't like it. The next taste, or another try the next day or week, may be accepted enthusiastically, perhaps because the strange taste is now familiar.	legumes, such as white beans, pinto beans, and black-eyed peas, cooked very soft or canned (rinse well) tropical fruits, cooked and pureed or mashed: pineapple, guava, kiwi, mango, papaya egg yolks cottage cheese, mashed grated cheddar, mozzarella, and Swiss cheeses cooked and finely minced chicken, turkey, white fish (check carefully for small bones), and beef pasta, well cooked and cut into small pieces soft tofu, mashed
At eight to ten months Your baby is now able to eat many table foods. You will be continually surprised at what	most cooked fruits and vegetables are O.K. now raw, peeled, diced fresh tomatoes

BABY'S AGE	FOODS TO TRY
his gums can "chew," but don't press your luck by giving him huge pieces of things, especially if he tends to gulp down food without carefully picking it apart first (babies, like people, have different styles of eating). He is still learning about chewing and swallowing, so keep food cut to a size he can handle. He may want nothing but finger food during this time because he is so pleased that he can feed himself. This desire is easily accommodated, and the practice is good for him. Once the novelty wears off, he'll probably let you feed him again and/or be ready to try using a spoon himself.	raw, diced pineapple and citrus fruits (remove seeds and tough white membranes)
At ten to twelve months By this age, your baby is pretty much able to eat what you eat, providing what you eat is healthy, primarily sugar-, salt-, and additive-free, and cooked well enough to be mashed with sturdy gums. If you haven't already, try offering her a spoon and a bowl of food (the bowls with suction-cup bottoms are handy, until she figures out how	whole eggs, scrambled or made into omelets and cut into strips (check with your doctor first) creamy peanut butter, good to spread on toast and cut into cubes (check with your doctor first about this nut product) tofu, cubed

BABY'S AGE	FOODS TO TRY
to break the suction and toss the bowl on the floor anyway). The new game of figuring out how to work utensils will probably fascinate her for quite some time, and you, so recently eager to start spoon-feeding your baby, will be glad for the break.	most healthy table foods, cut to manageable size

DANGER FOODS!

Honey can contain botulism spores, which a young system can't handle. Do not give your baby anything containing honey until he is at least one year old.

Avoid giving your baby the following foods, which are all serious choking hazards, until your child has all her teeth and is a competent chewer, at three or four years old. Many parents give babies a whole carrot to chew on when they are teething, but this is a big mistake. A baby can bite off a big chunk and choke before you realize what has happened.

- hot dogs (the number one cause of choking death in toddlers)
- nuts
- popcorn
- whole grapes
- ice cubes or chips
- hard candy
- raw carrots

FATHER ALERT!

IT'S YOUR TURN NOW

For the father eager to participate in feeding his child, now is the time! Meals can become a great bonding experience for you and your baby, and you may be the best person to begin introducing solids because you don't have those tempting breasts to distract the baby from the task at hand. Patience is in order, however. Eating is a complicated business and it takes a while to master. If you can be there to help your baby through it, you will always cherish the memories (made more vivid by the stains on your clothing!).

For the not-so-eager father, remember that Mom has put in an extreme amount of time feeding your baby up to this point. Reciprocation now will mean gratitude from your partner and a new facet of your relationship with your baby, who is getting more interesting every day. Try it and you'll probably be glad for the experience.

bond. When the breastfeeding relationship ends, your baby will still need your love, support, guidance, and physical presence for many years to come. Rather than mourning the loss of your infant, revel in your toddler's growth, reinforce your child's accomplishments, and begin the exciting process of building self-esteem, independence, and character. The old saying is true: Your child will always be your baby.

FEEDING THE BABY

As soon as she is ready, let the baby feed herself. When your baby starts grabbing for the spoon and is swallowing well, usually

IF YOUR BABY IS CHOKING

- ◎ Lay your baby facedown along your forearm at an angle with her head toward the floor, supporting her head and shoulders on your hand.

- ◎ Deliver five sharp blows with the palm of your other hand between her shoulder blades. (But not hard enough to cause further injury!)

- ◎ If she continues to choke, turn her faceup on your other arm with her head angled down, place two fingers on the lower half of her breastbone, and deliver five sharp downward (toward her head) thrusts, which imitate the action of a cough.

- ◎ Look in her mouth, putting your finger on her tongue so you can see the throat. Do not stick your finger in her mouth unless you can clearly see the obstruction and hook it out. Otherwise, you may lodge the obstruction more firmly in her throat.

- ◎ If she still can't breathe, call 911 immediately, then repeat the entire process until help arrives.

- ◎ IF YOUR BABY LOSES CONSCIOUSNESS, you must resuscitate her. Learn how to perform infant resuscitation, which may include mouth-to-mouth breathing and/or cardiopulmonary resuscitation (CPR).

We sincerely hope your baby never has to experience choking or resuscitation, but knowledge is everything in an emergency situation. An excellent book to buy and keep readily available in your home is the Johns Hopkins Children's Center's *First Aid for Children Fast,* which demonstrates emergency medical care for all common emergencies with simple instructions and excellent photographs. Buy it, or a similar book, today.

around six to eight months, she is probably ready to try finger foods. Your life will become even easier at this point. You can actually put the food right on her high chair tray and let her eat it herself! No more monotonous shoveling. Simply give your baby well-cooked or soft foods you had been pureeing, but chopped into small bites. Watch her carefully and never let her eat finger foods unsupervised or while walking around or lying down. She needs time to learn how to chew and swallow, and a baby's gag reflex isn't as strong as an adult's.

Choking and Choking Hazards

Before you start giving your baby finger foods, talk to your doctor about signing up for a CPR class (new fathers should do this too) that includes instruction for resuscitating infants, toddlers, and small children, and in administering cardiopulmonary resuscitation. It may be the most important class you ever take.

If your baby does start to choke, *do not* intervene as long as she is coughing, gagging, and making noise. Slapping her on the back or putting your finger in her mouth can make it worse. Coughing and gagging means her body is dislodging the food itself. However, if she stops breathing, turns blue, and cannot make any noise, she is choking and you *should* intervene.

Choking fears aside, don't be alarmed by occasional gagging. Gagging is a part of the learning process, and gives a baby a chance to learn what can be swallowed and what must be chewed. On the other hand, don't give your baby pieces of food too big to handle, or anything that can't be gummed, until he has grown in molars.

Buying Baby Food

Jars of baby food can be convenient for traveling or when you just don't have anything else on hand. Buy baby food carefully,

BABY FOOD IN DISGUISE

Some foods make great baby foods even though they aren't in the baby food aisle of the supermarket. These foods require little if any preparation and are truly convenient, inexpensive, and nutritious. Keep your refrigerator and pantry stocked with them at all times.

- unsweetened applesauce
- canned pumpkin
- plain yogurt
- cottage cheese (low salt), mashed
- oatmeal
- grits
- dehydrated mashed potatoes
- ripe bananas, mashed
- very ripe or canned (without sugar) peaches and pears, mashed

however. Read the labels; choose organic baby foods if they are available. Never buy baby food with added salt, sugar, starch, or other unnecessary ingredients. Buy basic, single-ingredient foods and mix a meat and a vegetable, say, or add a fruit to plain yogurt (once your baby has tried each food on his own). Baby food "meals" tend to have more additives and tend to be filled primarily with the cheapest ingredients (for instance, a chicken vegetable dinner may have hardly any chicken—check the protein content and the order of ingredients).

Making Your Own Baby Food

Making your own baby food may sound like something for mothers with nothing else to do (*are* there such mothers?). However, you can raise your baby without ever buying one single little glass jar of baby food. The trick is to make baby food in batches and in tandem with grown-up food, and use that freezer!

Your most valuable allies, if you plan to feed your baby in this way, will be your freezer, your blender, and your microwave. (Even the microwave is optional.) Cooking for your family can be a fun and creative endeavor, without having to be time-consuming. Every recipe in the "Mini Family Cookbook" you'll find at the back of this book is simple and fast to prepare, as well as being delicious for your baby and for you.

6

❦ BARRIERS TO BREASTFEEDING SUCCESS

♪TRIKE BACK AT A NURSING STRIKE!

W HEN your baby suddenly refuses to nurse and is too young to wean, you are probably experiencing a nursing strike, and figuring out the cause can be a frustrating process. When you try to nurse, your baby may cry, bite you, turn away, even push you away. Do not feel personally rejected by this behavior. Instead, figure out what is wrong.

If your baby is younger than twelve months—and even more importantly, if he is under nine months—a nursing strike does *not* mean he is ready to wean, although weaning is often the result because, unable to find the cause, Mom gives up and "accepts" the end of nursing. Your infant will benefit immensely from a full year of nursing, so you will both be better off if you get to the bottom of the nursing strike instead of letting it get the better of you.

If your baby won't nurse, examine her physical state. Is she comfortable? Is anything hurting her? Is she teething, or does she have something wrong with her mouth such as a cut, a sore, or thrush (an oral yeast infection, see page 153)? If everything seems fine physically, take a good look at your environment and your attitude. Are any major changes taking place in your household? Have you become distracted while nursing? Are you engaged in any sort of behavior while nursing that might frighten or confuse your baby, such as disciplining other children, talking loudly on the phone, or trying to get things done simultaneously? Are you experiencing marital, financial, or work-related difficulties? If so, you need to take special care while nursing to put your worries and distractions aside. Nurse your baby in a quiet, calm location, away from the fray of daily life.

Resolving a nursing strike is important—your milk supply diminishes during a strike but can usually be reestablished with a little attention. It's a Catch 22: the nursing strike causes your milk supply to diminish, which in turn makes it harder for your baby to get enough milk, which precipitates weaning. Pump breastmilk during a nursing strike if you need to, to ease engorgement and keep your milk supply flowing while you use your powers of determination to get back on track; but never stop offering your breast. Try not to let the temporary inconvenience of a nursing strike lead you to give up nursing. Remember the wonderful benefits of breastmilk for your baby and stick with it.

When you, your baby, or any other family member gets sick, the breastfeeding life may suffer, or at least feel the effects. Preventing sickness in your household is the ideal remedy, but when someone gets a cold, the flu, an ear infection, thrush, or something worse, you will have to deal with it. Luckily, the breastfeeding infant will be largely protected from illnesses to which you are exposed (remember from chapter 1 that you pass on antibodies through your breastmilk that help protect the baby), so even if you have a cold or the flu—*especially* when you have a cold or the flu—you should continue to breastfeed. Limit the kissing, but keep up the nursing.

Knowing when to call the doctor is important. Many minor illnesses don't require a doctor's care, but certain conditions definitely do. If you are ever in any doubt about whether to call the doctor or not, call. Doctors are there to help you, no matter what time of day it is. Trust your instincts. If you feel something serious is wrong with your baby or any other family member, call, even if it is at night or on a weekend.

Here are some of the most common causes of nursing strikes and problems, and what you can do about them.

⟣ TEETHING (OUCH!) ⟢

Although some babies barely notice when their teeth emerge and some turn to nursing for comfort when teething, others seem to feel considerable pain. Teething generally begins around six months, but varies widely among infants. Signs that teething may be starting include excessive drooling, chapped skin on the baby's chin (caused by drooling), gagging and coughing, crankiness, and, yes, gnawing and biting you.

Sensitive gums can make nursing uncomfortable, and your baby may turn away, cry, or bite you (the pressure of biting can feel good on sore gums). If the problem persists or seems very serious—your baby won't eat, for example—talk to your doctor about teething remedies. You may notice that your baby will show a constant urge to nurse, followed by rejection of the breast shortly after nursing starts because the pain of teething is exacerbated by the sucking reflex. This can be frustrating for both members of the nursing couple. Resourcefulness and patience are the key to getting through the teething period.

Here are some teething strategies you can try at home. Rub his gums with your finger (wash your hands first with disinfectant soap), give him teething rings chilled in the freezer (but don't hang teething rings around his neck; that can cause strangulation), or give him a cold, wet washcloth for gnawing. Experiment with different nursing positions, which may feel different to him and be more successful. Stay relaxed and reassuring. He may be confused by the pain and will need extra love and comforting, which you can also offer without nursing. Once a particular problem tooth emerges, the pain may lessen, so keep trying. Continually offering the breast is important because even if he doesn't want to nurse on a few occasions, you don't want him to associate his pain with any separation from you. If you are worried about the baby's fluid intake, offer additional fluids, such as water or juice (with your pediatrician's okay) in a cup or bottle. Chilling the beverage can also help relieve teething pain. Try feeding him chilled soft foods, such as applesauce or mashed fruits, if he's starting on solids. Biting a cup rim, bottle nipple, pacifier or spoon may also offer relief.

Avoid giving your baby hard food to bite on to relieve teething pain, such as a raw carrot or frozen bagel, as are commonly recommended; even though he doesn't have many teeth now, he soon will and he'll expect you to continue to give him raw carrots, etc., to chew on. Hard foods such as carrots are a serious choking hazard! Try a chilled (not frozen) banana slice instead, which can be gummed down to a soft mush as it warms up in his mouth.

As your baby's teeth come in, she will want to try them out, and that includes during nursing. This isn't a violent gesture, but a natural one. She'll bite on anything that crosses her path—from crib rails to her own fingers. If she bites you while nursing, a sharp "no" will probably scare her, and her look of surprise might make you laugh. *Don't laugh*. The baby will be confused by your mixed message—a sharp tone followed by laughter—and she'll likely hope your laughter means you think her biting is funny, which could elicit more biting. Try this behavioral strategy to stop biting from becoming habit-forming while nursing: Say "no" firmly (but not threateningly), take your baby away from the breast temporarily, and look at her with a serious expression. She might cry, but she will get the message, if not the first time, after a time or two. Most importantly, don't get angry at your baby. She isn't trying to hurt you. But do nip biting in the bud.

Don't let the teething phase prompt weaning if you aren't otherwise ready. Your infant will soon learn that biting means no breast, and he will keep his teeth to himself, at least while nursing. A similar response to biting your finger, shoulder, or the dog's ear will be similarly effective: a firm "no," a quick separation of baby and victim, and a serious expression. Biting is a stage most babies experience, and it does not mean they are ready to wean. Remember that your baby is receiving all the nutritious and immune-boosting benefits of your milk as long as he nurses. A few teeth aren't any reason to deny him of those benefits. Yes, biting hurts, but you'll live—and this is an opportunity to teach.

To relieve any soreness or chafing to your nipples during this teething stage, try rubbing a bit of vegetable oil onto them. Or apply aloe vera gel right after nursing and wash it off right before you nurse again, if it hasn't been fully absorbed. Your baby's teething probably won't break the skin—that's more likely to occur from chafing and chapping, when the skin cracks. In either case, you might also want to put some antibiotic ointment on your nipples, but very lightly, only once a day, and be sure it is completely absorbed or washed off before you nurse again. This will help to head off any possible infection, though remember that your Montgomery glands should take care of this very nicely in most cases—ask your doctor for advice if you think you might need to use an antibiotic cream.

If nursing is painful for you and/or your baby but he doesn't seem to be teething, the culprit may be thrush (see page 153).

THE COMMON COLD

If your little one has a stuffy nose, she won't be able to breathe well while nursing. If she shows signs of a mild cold, such as coughing, a runny nose, sniffling and sneezing, fussiness, and a low-grade fever (under 101 degrees Fahrenheit), you probably don't need a doctor *unless it's her first cold or she is under four months old*, but you may need to help relieve her congestion so she can nurse easily. Try suctioning her nose with a bulb syringe. A little warm salt water in her nose will often loosen stuffiness and facilitate draining (mix one-quarter teaspoon salt in a cup of lukewarm water to prepare the saline solution or buy saline drops). If she won't let you get the syringe near her nose, cup some salt water in your hand and gently pat it against her nostrils (but don't hold it there or splash her in the face). Also, run a humidifier in the baby's room to help her decongest; a few drops of eucalyptus oil in the water will be soothing (do not apply the oil directly to your child's skin, however, and *never* give or take it internally). Nurse the baby often. A gentle chest massage can also help to break up congestion.

If your baby has breathing difficulty that is not relieved by suctioning the nose, if she seems extremely upset or in pain, if she's increasingly lethargic, if she refuses to eat or nurse, or if she has a dry cough that lasts longer than two weeks, call the doctor and schedule an appointment immediately. The symptoms of a cold are similar to those of allergies, the flu, and chicken pox (your baby can be infected with the virus that causes chicken pox through exposure to an older child). To help prevent colds from spreading, all family members should wash their hands regularly with disinfectant soap, especially before touching or holding the baby.

For children over one year old, warm water with a small pinch of ginger, the juice of half a lemon, and two teaspoons of honey can be very soothing and can be repeated every few hours; the honey acts as a natural cough suppressant (*never* give honey to a child under one year of age—it can contain botulism spores). You might want to try this remedy yourself, if you are the one with the cold. Other good natural remedies for nursing mothers with colds include peppermint tea to bring down a fever and gargling a saline solution of one teaspoon salt in one cup of warm water to ease a sore throat. Fruit sherbert, cold yogurt, or a fresh fruit smoothie (see the Mini Family Cookbook on page 245) can feel great on a sore throat, too.

THE FLU

Like colds, influenza is spread by human contact, from coughing and sneezing or through touch. Influenza cases are often most severe in people with developing immune systems, such as infants, or in those with impaired immune systems, such as the elderly or chronically ill. Suggest that grandparents and elderly or ill people who may come into contact with your child receive yearly anti-influenza immunizations to reduce the risk of spreading infection to your baby. If they don't, refrain from allowing them to hold your infant. These immunizations generally are not administered to infants under six months as there hasn't been enough study of the risks and benefits of doing so.

If your baby is having frequent vomiting and/or diarrhea (after every feeding, or to the extent that the baby is becoming dehydrated, with decreased urine output), or is experiencing a fever over 101 degrees F (from birth to four months) or over 103 degrees F (for babies over four months) associated with the flu, call your doctor immediately. Continue breastfeeding. Your pediatrician may also suggest supplementing breastmilk with Pedialyte for infants or fruit juices or sports drinks for older babies. Antibiotics are not effective against cold or flu viruses and should be avoided. Remember that if you've been exposed to the same flu virus your baby has contracted, your breastmilk will pass on virus-fighting antibodies, so your milk will have both a nourishing *and* a medicinal effect on the baby.

Several acupressure points on the foot, according to some, can ease the symptoms of fever, achiness, and stomach distress which often accompany the flu (for both nursing mothers and babies who come down with it). Try a gentle foot massage: Rotate each toe, press into the center of each toe for a few seconds, press directly under the big toe and hold, massage the ball of each foot, make thumbprints across the bottom of the foot from the midline to the ball, and make small circles around the anklebones of each foot, pressing into any tender points until they become less tender.

Nursing mothers who have the flu need to be careful to stay hydrated. Drink fruit juices, ginger ale, or an electrolyte-rich sports drink to keep fluid levels high for breastfeeding. But before taking any kind of medication to control flu symptoms, over-the-

FEVERS, BREASTFEEDING, AND REYE'S SYNDROME

When your baby has a fever, it is important to continue breastfeeding as normally as possible to keep his intake of fluids high enough to prevent dehydration (especially if the fever is accompanied by diarrhea or vomiting). Your milk is the most superior food for him during any illness. Electrolyte fluids, such as Pedialyte, should be used as *supplements* to breastfeeding, if necessary. Sponge him with cool water and allow the skin to dry naturally as the water evaporates. Dress him in loose, light clothing and cover with light blankets.

Fevers of 101 degrees F or more are considered serious in infants of four months or younger, 103 degrees or more in older babies. If your baby has a fever in this range, you'll want to call the doctor immediately.

IMPORTANT: *Never* give your baby aspirin to ward off a fever. Aspirin given to children under fifteen has been linked to an acute, life-threatening disorder called Reye's syndrome, the cause of which is unknown. Consult your physician for advice on the proper analgesic (pain-killing), fever-reducing agent; acetaminophen in infant or child dosages (one brand is Children's Tylenol) is usually recommended.

counter or otherwise, consult your physician. If you are having trouble keeping anything down, take in no food or liquid for two hours after vomiting, then try a spoonful of clear liquid (the choices above are good ones) every fifteen minutes. If this stays down, after an hour increase to two spoonfuls every fifteen minutes. If this is successful for several hours, very bland food (dry toast, apple sauce, oatmeal) can be tried. Keep nursing the baby. Take special care to wash your hands with disinfectant soap before nursing and to avoid coughing or sneezing in his direction—you don't want this flu virus to hang around any longer than it has to! (And no kissing!)

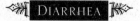

DIARRHEA

Your baby's diarrhea can be caused by food allergies or it can be a sign of gastroenteritis, a serious condition requiring immediately attention from your pediatrician. Frequent (more than his usual pattern) loose, runny stools indicate diarrhea. In most cases, mothers should continue to nurse throughout an episode of infant diarrhea and, perhaps, supplement breastmilk with clear fluids, such as Pedialyte. Baby will be reassured by the familiar comfort of nursing, and breastmilk is much better tolerated by infants with diarrhea than formula is. In fact, a 1995 study at Johns Hopkins Children's Center reveals that mucin, a protein in breastmilk, suppresses the reproduction of rotavirus, a primary cause of diarrhea in infants. Other substances in breastmilk may also contribute to a decreased risk of intestinal disorders and studies are under way to find out more.

If diarrhea is persistent and severe, however, even breastmilk may be difficult for him to digest. During this time, breastfeeding may be temporarily interrupted, so you'll want to pump milk to keep your supply from diminishing and ensure that you'll be able to begin breastfeeding with no problem when he's feeling better.

Too much sugar in a baby's diet can cause diarrhea. Avoid giving him fruit juices sweetened with sugar and stick to all-natural varieties that have been pasteurized, cut with one-half spring water. Also, if you've introduced solids too quickly and your baby isn't ready for them, diarrhea may result. For older babies, sugar syrup–based medications may be the cause of diarrhea; continue administering the medication but contact your physician to see if a different drug can be substituted. Antibiotics taken by you can also aggravate his digestive system, as can iron supplements you take (see chapter 5). But don't try to diagnose the cause of diarrhea yourself—that's your pediatrician's job.

If diarrhea persists more than twenty-four hours or is accompanied by vomiting or a high fever, if blood is present in baby's stool, or if he shows signs of dehydration (such as decreased urine output), contact your doctor as soon as possible. Dehydration associated with diarrhea can be a life-threatening condition in babies. Other signs of dehyration include no tears when crying, sunken fontanel (a depressed spot on the top of the baby's head), dry mouth, dry or wrinkled skin, dark urine, and sunken eyes.

VOMITING

First you'll need to make the distinction between spitting up, the normal process of regurgitation, and vomiting. As we noted in chapter 4, some babies are just Spit-Up Artists. Even isolated incidents of vomiting (or diarrhea) are usually nothing to worry about. If your baby has two or three wet diapers a day during a period of illness, such as a cold, there's no great risk of dehydration. If she's having trouble keeping anything down, though, try smaller, more frequent feedings. Remember that breastmilk is the substance most easily digested by a baby and even if she doesn't keep all of it down, many of the nutrients and fluids in your milk will be absorbed immediately. You might want to express some milk for future use (see "Expressing Breastmilk Manually" on page 56 or "Breast Pump Choices" on page 91) and allow her to nurse from a partially empty breast. If she's over six months and has started on solids, you'll want to withdraw the solids and give only breastmilk until her stomach settles down. Don't forget: continuing to nurse provides nourishment *and* comfort to your little one. The familiar closeness of breastfeeding will calm and reassure you both.

If your baby vomits after every breastfeeding session for a six-hour period and/or the vomiting is accompanied by high fever or diarrhea, call your physician immediately to avoid the potential for life-threatening dehydration.

FAMILY ALERT!

ASEPTIC HANDWASH FOR "INFECTION CONTROL"

Aseptic handwash is a technique that health care professionals use routinely to ensure good hygiene and to control the potential spread of infectious illness. Your new family should get into the habit of using this handwashing method on a regular basis. Here's what you do:

◉ Remove all jewelry (rings can harbor microorganisms). Place a role of paper towels nearby. It's a good idea to install a wall dispenser for paper towels in the bathroom, so that you have easy access to clean towels that aren't touching potentially contaminated sinks or other surfaces.

◉ Remove a paper towel from the dispenser and use it to turn on the faucet without directly touching the hardware. Discard the used paper towel. Place your hands under the lukewarm running water, immersing them completely. Avoid touching the sides of the sink.

◉ Apply disinfectant soap and scrub by rubbing your hands together and reaching between each finger.

◉ Use a nail brush to clean under the nails.

◉ Rinse hands thoroughly under running water, again reaching between the fingers. Keep your hands pointed down and hold them lower than your elbows; this allows the "contaminated" water to run into the sink and not up onto your forearms.

◉ Use a paper towel to dry your hands and then use the same paper towel to turn off the faucet without touching it directly with your hands. Discard the used paper towel without touching the waste can.

You can boost the effectiveness of aseptic handwashing by regularly cleaning bathroom and kitchen surfaces (especially faucet handles) and all doorknobs and handles (especially the bathroom) when a family member is ill. Of course, anyone who touches or holds your baby should wash his or her hands first, if possible.

Another way to limit your child's exposure to pathogens is to change her diaper regularly, and more frequently during a bout of illness. Moisture draws bacteria and encourages its growth.

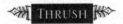

THRUSH

If your baby suddenly seems to have trouble latching on or acts unusually fussy when nursing, and/or if you experience sudden painful nipple soreness when nursing, thrush may be the culprit. Thrush is essentially a yeast infection in your baby's mouth. A baby's first opportunity to come into contact with yeast is during birth, as most pregnant women have some amount of yeast in their vaginas. Yeast, the fungus *Candida albicans,* is common in everyone's body and only poses a problem when it overgrows. Thrush is particularly common if your baby has been on antibiotics (which kill the bacteria that keep yeast in check), during the summer months, and in hot, humid climates (which encourage yeast growth). If he isn't teething but nursing seems painful, look inside his mouth. Thrush looks like a white, cheesy substance or spit-up milk on the insides of your baby's cheeks or on his tongue, but it won't wipe away. Many cases of thrush will resolve themselves, but if he has a bad case, your doctor may prescribe an anti-fungal agent to help get rid of it faster. Yeast may also cause diaper rash (red, raised bumps on a baby's bottom), so thrush and diaper rash often occur simultaneously. Thrush-induced diaper rash is best treated with an anti-fungal creme your doctor can prescribe.

To help prevent diaper rash, always clean the baby's bottom thoroughly when you change her diaper, and in the presence of diaper rash, don't use diaper wipes. A paper towel or soft cloth and plain water is less irritating. Also, before rediapering, aim a blow dryer *on low cool only* about six inches away from the baby's bottom. Change her diaper frequently so sensitive skin is usually in contact with a dry diaper—even getting up to change your sleeping baby's diaper. If the weather is humid, use a cornstarch-based baby powder (talc can be harmful when inhaled by your baby). If diaper rash is already present, avoid putting tight-fitting clothes or plastic pants on your baby's bottom. Zinc oxide cream (such as Desitin) will keep the rash dry. If weather permits, let your child sit or run around outside in the buff—the fresh air and sunshine can help dry out the rash. If diaper rash or thrush persists longer than two weeks (or less if it seems to be bothering either the baby or you), call your doctor.

If you've got thrush on your nipples, they'll become red, sore, and, sometimes, cracked. Nursing may become quite painful for you. To try to avoid getting infected with your baby's case of thrush, air dry your nipples after each breastfeeding session. If you do become infected with thrush, anti-fungal cremes (such as Lotrimin) are the best remedy, but be sure the creme is fully absorbed or washed off before nursing. Some doctors may recommend gentian violet, a dark purple liquid that stains everything it touches and is therefore often more trouble than it is worth. You may also find that you develop a vaginal yeast infection, which is caused by the same fungus, *Candida albicans*.

Thrush can be difficult to cure, especially in the summer or in warm, humid climates, but it isn't harmful, just irritating. If you

FATHER ALERT!

HELP YOUR NURSING COUPLE BREAK DOWN BARRIERS

Nursing problems may leave you feeling confused, frustrated, and helpless as you watch your partner and baby struggle to get their breastfeeding relationship back on track. You *can* help by providing much-needed support and comfort. Cuddle and reassure the baby. If he's sick, offer to sit with him or to administer medications so your partner can get a break from round-the-clock care. Show a willingness to discuss nursing challenges with your partner and encourage her to seek help if ready solutions aren't available or don't seem to be working. Make sure the whole family practices stress-management techniques, such as those outlined in chapter 7. Above all, let your nursing couple know that you support the decision to stick with breastfeeding, for as long as they want to keep with it. Remember that positive reinforcement is far more beneficial than negative messages— praise your partner's efforts to continue breastfeeding and remind her of the great gift she's already given your baby through the time you and she, as a new parent team, have already devoted to the breastfeeding life.

both get thrush, wash your bras frequently, use disposable nursing pads, and boil all teethers, pacifiers, bottle nipples, and toys that have come into contact with your baby's mouth. High sugar diets (yours or your baby's) may encourage excessive yeast. If you can't get rid of thrush, try cutting out all refined sugar from your diet and increasing your (and your baby's) intake of plain yogurt, which is rich in the good bacteria that control yeast (look for yogurt that contains live, active cultures). Avoid flavored yogurts, which contain too much sugar. You can even apply plain yogurt to the baby's diaper rash and your nipples as well. The pain and irritation of thrush can cause both of you to want to give up on nursing, so resolve thrush as soon as possible and keep all her toys, teethers, bottles, and anything else in contact with her mouth scrupulously clean to avoid reinfection. All family members should wash their hands with disinfectant soap (including you) before touching or holding the baby.

Through it all, keep nursing. If your nipples become infected, contact your doctor immediately to begin treatment—*before* your nipples feel too sore to persist with nursing; you don't want to experience the diminished milk supply that accompanies a stop in nursing, which in turn can lead to premature weaning, and thrush can make pumping painful, too.

EARACHES (OTITIS MEDIA)

Babies who are breastfed for three months or more are far less likely to suffer from ear infections than bottle-fed babies. Otitis media is an infection of the middle ear that causes painful inflammation; babies are more prone to it than adults because their eustachian tubes are short and narrow. If your breastfed baby does get an ear infection, breastfeeding may be affected because the nerve that runs from the ear to the throat will radiate the pain of an earache to his jaw; sucking will make the pain of an earache more acute. Signs of an earache include ear pulling or rubbing, fever, irritability and crying, vomiting, and loss of appetite. Earaches are sometimes caused by nursing a baby in a prone position; milk can drain into the eustachian tube and become trapped, causing infection and inflammation. If your baby is predisposed to ear infections, try nursing him in sitting positions, or so that his head is at least slightly elevated. Ear infections are most painful for babies during the night, when they are lying flat; try placing a pillow under the baby's mattress to elevate his head a bit while sleeping. Your doctor may suggest baby acetaminophen, ear drops, and antibiotics to treat the otitis media. In severe cases, your baby may require ear tubes.

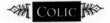

A colicky baby can be almost as distressing to new parents as she is to herself! Although there are many theories on the causes of colic, including an immature digestive system or the effect of overstimulation on an immature nervous system, its primary symptom is extended, intense crying, often accompanied by arching the body or flexing the knees toward the abdomen. Mysteriously, colic attacks are more common during the dinner hour. In some babies, relief seems impossible, but here are a few things to try:

◎ *Burp her periodically while feeding, and do not overfeed. Nursing more often with smaller feedings may help. Try holding her in an upright position for a while after feeding.*

◎ *Keep the household environment as calm and soothing as possible, eliminating sources of loud noise, stimulation, and tension (all common when everyone returns home at the end of the workday and prepares for dinner—perhaps a reason why colic often occurs at this time).*

◎ *Keep her warm (but not hot).*

◎ *When breastfeeding, try eliminating certain foods in your own diet, especially milk or foods that cause you gastric distress. She may have an allergic reaction to the cow's milk you are drinking.*

◎ *If you have recently introduced solid foods, go back to breastfeeding for a while, then carefully introduce a new food only about once a week.*

◎ *Make sure food is room temperature, not too cold.*

◉ *Rhythmic movement such as rocking, holding a vibrating pillow, or bouncing her on your chest while humming or singing might help (new fathers are often great at the latter).*

◉ *Try an infant massage, concentrating on rubbing the tummy gently with warm sesame oil (or other vegetable oil) and flexing the knees toward the abdomen (see chapter 7 for more on infant massage technique).*

◉ *Give plenty of cuddling and comfort. She'll be reassured to have you near until her episode of colic has passed.*

ALLERGIES

Your baby will never have an allergic reaction to breastmilk, his natural source of nutrition. In fact, the length of time you breastfeed has been shown to be directly related to your child's tendency to develop allergies as he grows up; babies who are breastfed the longest have the fewest allergies as children and adults. He may, however, be allergic to the protein in any cow's milk *you* may drink and in formulas based on cow's milk. If so, you'll want to switch to calcium-fortified soy milk for you and soy-based formulas for the baby, if his diet requires formula supplementation for any reason. If he's started on solid foods and begins to exhibit the signs of an allergic reaction, withdraw solids temporarily and breastfeed only. Take note of what he'd been eating and consult your physician about the possibility of a food allergy.

PHYSICAL CHANGES IN YOU

Certain strong foods you eat, such as garlic, may slightly alter the taste of your milk. If you begin menstruation while still nursing, your milk's taste may change slightly while you are menstruating. (Menstruation usually commences during the period of partial weaning. See chapter 10.) Babies are sensitive (some more than others), and any change in taste or smell might temporarily surprise them, making them refuse the breast. If you become pregnant again while nursing your older baby or toddler, this may affect the taste of your milk, too.

Also, any change in perfumes, lotions, deodorants/antiperspirants, or soaps may even be detectable and disturbing to your sensitive baby, precipitating a nursing strike. Cornstarch is a safe, effective substitute for deodorant or antiperspirant that may be causing trouble.

EXTERNAL DISTRACTIONS

Maybe you are distracted when nursing, not paying attention to your baby, or trying to rush her to finish. Maybe you are paying attention to your other children or the family pet while trying to nurse simultaneously. Maybe a loud television, a new environment, or the sounds of new people are distracting your sensitive baby. If she is used to quiet, undisturbed nursing, a new situation such as house guests or a move to a different house can be very distracting. If she has quit nursing and you have eliminated physical problems, examine the nursing environment. Once your baby is assured you are there for her no matter what else is going on, she will most likely be happily relieved to resume nursing.

If slow let-down is a problem for a successful start to nursing sessions, try expressing a little milk *before* you begin nursing. This will ensure that she tastes the milk right away and doesn't have to suck with no happy result (everyone loves instant gratification!). It can take as long as five minutes for your milk to flow freely.

STRESS
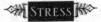

The mind is an amazing thing. It can be your most powerful ally in maintaining or regaining your health. It can also be your worst enemy. Your body responds to stress, and the breastfeeding body is particularly vulnerable. Although stress can be a positive force in life, spurring you into action, enhancing your joy, and pushing you to the peak of performance, it can also have a number of alarming effects on the breastfeeding life. However, the presence of stress should not discourage you from breastfeeding, nor should it precipitate weaning. In fact, stressful times are the worst times to consider weaning. The best way to assure your baby that everything is okay is through the familiar comfort of nursing. The best way for you to stay relatively stress-free is, first, to practice stress prevention; second, to be on the lookout for signs that stress is taking its toll; and third, to master the fine art of stress management. Stress as a barrier to breastfeeding success is such a large topic that we gave it its own chapter. See chapter 7 for everything you need to know about stress and the breastfeeding life.

SERIOUS ILLNESS IN YOUR FAMILY

We sincerely hope your family never has to deal with a more serious illness or accident, but some families inevitably will. Cancer, heart disease, stroke, diabetes, multiple sclerosis, mental illness (such as depression or schizophrenia), and many other major medical problems are an unfortunate reality for many families. A serious illness in mother or baby may not preclude breastfeeding, but you will need to discuss this with your doctor.

If illness is a major part of your family's life, optimism and hope can be difficult to maintain. Stress will be unavoidable and may, at times, seem insurmountable. Finding a support group of people with similar problems can be an incredible outlet and relief for many. Make sure, too, that you are satisfied with the medical care you are receiving. Learn as much as you can about your (or your child's) illness, and request that your doctor keep you as informed as possible about all aspects of your care. Knowledge is power.

THE POWER OF A POSITIVE ATTITUDE

With effort, patience, and a little time, almost every barrier to breastfeeding can be overcome. If you are struggling with a breastfeeding problem or nursing strike, feel overwhelmed by your situation, or are afraid you may have no choice but to abandon the breastfeeding relationship, seek help immediately from your health care team, your family, a local support group of breastfeeding mothers, a certified lactation consultant, or the La Leche League. In other words, find somebody out there who is compassionate, knowledgeable, and ready to assist you. Help exists! You and your new family are not alone. Like any other relationship in your life, the breastfeeding relationship requires care and attention in both the easy times and the rough times. Whether you breastfeed for two weeks, six months, a year, or more, your time is rewarded through the rich health benefits you've given to your child, the handsome payoff of the breastfeeding life. Try to keep the breastfeeding relationship going for as long as you and your baby want it to; premature weaning is unnecessary for most nursing couples.

As you face breastfeeding challenges, keep a positive attitude and focus on finding workable solutions, instead of becoming stressed out and letting the situation get the better of you. Make a conscious effort to focus on the loving bond you share with your child while nursing. Relax. Smile. You are teaching your child the virtues of persistence, resilience, and determination, not to mention good health and how to overcome adversity with loving support. These are pretty good accomplishments for the first year of life. Give your little one a cuddle for us.

7

STRESSBUSTERS FOR THE BREASTFEEDING LIFE

Stress, Stress, and More Stress!

STRESS isn't good for you, but as an adult, you are used to it. Your baby, on the other hand, hasn't developed your repertoire of stress-defeating strategies. One of your jobs as a parent is to protect your infant from all types of harmful conditions, and stress can certainly be harmful. Of course, your baby will be able to detect any negative feelings you are experiencing, so part of this job involves keeping yourself and your family relatively stress-free.

Your baby may show signs of stress by being unusually fussy, refusing to eat, suddenly waking frequently at night when he had previously been sleeping through, losing weight, or generally seeming unhappy or not "right." (There are other causes for all of these symptoms, too. See chapter 6, "Barriers to Breastfeeding Success.") We cannot emphasize enough how important it is to be tuned in to your newest family member. Luckily, the breastfeeding mother is in direct contact with her baby frequently throughout the day. If you notice signs of stress in your baby's behavior, try immediately to determine the cause so you can fix it. If you can't figure it out, call your doctor.

Your family dynamic is the result of a complex interaction of forces. When any one of these forces is having a problem, the others will feel it. The best way to keep your family on an even keel is open, frequent communication. Each family member should continually monitor the rest of the family for stress overload. Don't let a single day go by without talking to and touching every single member of your family (pets included!). Every family member should spend some time each day touching and talking to the baby. It is easy to get so busy that you forget what is important. Life is short—so make the most of each precious moment of family life together; an important part of holistic living is keeping in touch.

OLDER SIBLINGS: THE GREAT COMPETITION

If this baby isn't the first and you have an older child or children in the house, sibling rivalry may create a stress-management challenge for the whole family. Consider how your older child feels. No longer the center of your world, she has been temporarily sidelined. She may love the new baby or she may be terribly jealous. Chances are, she is experiencing a combination of both feelings, which is very stressful and confusing for her, as well as for you and for other family members, who have to deal with her reactions, outbursts, attempts to regain the spotlight, even her aggression toward the new baby.

Use nursing time to reassure your older child. Let her snuggle with you and little baby brother and hold a book while you read it aloud and nurse your baby. Make a special activity box with crayons, paper dolls, small toys, or other items your child considers special, to be opened only when you are nursing the baby. Before you start to nurse, prepare a snack for your child and explain that she and her baby sibling are snacking together, but that she has the "big girl snack."

Also, recognize that your instincts will be to protect and lavish attention on your newborn. Your more self-sufficient child may get ignored, especially if she isn't very forward or demanding. Make a conscious effort to reassure her and, whenever possible, ask her to help you. Children love to participate in baby care if they are given a chance. Most importantly, remember to nurture her self-esteem, and she will become a loving sibling and reliable helper.

You may also experience feelings of guilt about not being able to give your first child as much attention as she once enjoyed. Don't overcompensate by giving in to your older child's every desire. Instead, help her to define her new role as an older sibling by teaching her that she can be increasingly independent, self-sufficient, and magnanimously unselfish, "like a big kid."

And one more great advantage to breastfeeding: bottle-feeding takes two hands, but nursing allows you a free hand to hold and cuddle your toddler. Let all your children participate in the breastfeeding life, each in his or her own way. If you are still nursing your toddler, tandem nursing of toddler and newborn can be used as a way to teach the older child social skills, such as sharing and cooperation, and can be used as a way to comfort and reassure. See chapter 10 for more information on tandem nursing. For those who have outgrown nursing, bring them into your circle. Let them nurture and gently touch the nursing baby. Hug them, talk to them, and let them pamper you, too. Tell them you need their help to get you a cool drink so you can nurse better, or to find you a good pillow for propping your arms or back.

Sometimes, of course, you will want and need to nurse your newborn alone. It's only fair to the new baby. Share some of your nursing sessions, but explain to older children that other sessions are just for the baby. Then be sure to set aside some time for other children to have you to themselves, too. If they aren't deprived of solo access to you, they'll be more willing to share you.

The bigger your family, the harder it will be to spend individual time with each child. However, making an effort to do so will go a long way toward fostering family harmony and closeness. All too soon, your children will be grown and setting out on adventures of their own! Cherish your family togetherness while

FATHER ALERT!

YOUR JOB AS STRESS POLICE

Both you and your partner will sometimes be overwhelmed by the stresses of your new parenting roles. You can help to support your breastfeeding team by working to alleviate stressful situations as best you can. If your partner becomes particularly irritable or frustrated, acts suddenly depressed or "low," seems withdrawn, changes her eating or sleeping habits suddenly, or just plain tells you she can't take it anymore, find ways to help her relax. Encourage her to talk about her feelings with you. Offer to take over some of her household duties for a while, or to spend more time with the new baby and/or older siblings. Let her get out of the house without the baby. Tell her what a great job she is doing. Spend quality time with your partner doing something you both enjoy—whether it's renting a video or getting a sitter for a dinner out. And when (or if) you feel super-stressed or ready to blow up, explain to your partner that you need some time out.

The important thing: make sure lines of communication are always kept open and that your conversations have adequate time and space to unfold. If you're trying to talk about stressful situations while you're both doing a hundred things, you'll only add to the stress! When you're too busy to talk, make an "appointment" to talk later. Make sure you both keep it.

And don't worry about feeling pressured to be "Super Dad." Who needs the stress? A *really* super dad is one who can admit he's only human (and that everyone else is too!) and who shows a willingness to solve stressful problems together as a family.

your children are growing, paying careful attention even to tantrum-throwing toddlers and tenacious teenagers. They all need love and support, just as much as your littlest one.

STRESS AND YOUR MILK SUPPLY

Your milk supply is self-regulating, in that it corresponds to your baby's demand. As your baby gets older and nurses less, your supply will gradually diminish. However, sometimes stress can subvert nature's normally well-orchestrated plan, prematurely causing a too-diminished supply. When you are feeling anxious, you may unintentionally inhibit the milk ejection reflex normally triggered by the prolactin surge caused by the baby's sucking, so it is important to relax and focus on your baby when nursing. Too many nursing sessions without the milk ejection reflex will cause your milk supply to diminish. Also, during extremely busy times, such as the holidays, you may actually nurse less often without realizing it. This could also result in a diminished milk supply. The best way to remedy this problem: consciously nurse more often, even if for short periods of time. Watch the clock, or even set a timer, if necessary. If your supply diminishes, your baby may become frustrated and refuse to nurse because milk isn't flowing freely or quickly enough. This in turn will diminish your supply further and may result in involuntary premature weaning (see page 142, "Strike Back at a Nursing Strike!").

If you suspect your milk supply has diminished before its time, nurse more often, focus completely on the nursing process while nursing, increase your fluid intake, and practice the stress management techniques outlined in this chapter. Your milk supply should replenish quickly.

POSTPARTUM BLUES

Many new mothers experience some degree of postpartum depression after giving birth. Some attribute this depression to changing hormonal levels, others to the profound realization that after childbirth, a new mother's life is unalterably changed. It may just be a little of both. And while breastfeeding mothers have the surge of prolactin to relax them and stimulate maternal feelings, they still experience the blues as frequently as mothers who bottle-feed their babies.

The introduction of a new baby into your family's life is a cause for great joy, but also for great change and adjustment to a new way of living. Your newborn requires round-the-clock care. And if you're breastfeeding, you'll be scheduling your day for the needs of two people—not just one (maybe even for three or more people, if you count your partner and any other children you already have!). Remember, too, that breastfeeding is a learned behavior for both mothers and babies. It may take time for breastfeeding to feel "natural" or "right" to you. For some nursing mothers, breastfeeding is never a fairy tale, earth mother experience, and this realization may spark feelings of stress or sadness at first—but that doesn't mean these mothers can't have successful breastfeeding relationships with their babies, or that they feel any less strongly about giving their babies the health benefits of breastfeeding. Different people respond differently; give yourself room to explore how you feel about breastfeeding—without judging your own emotions or being too hard on yourself if it takes some time to get used to the breastfeeding relationship.

New mothers are under enormous pressure, from both external and internal sources, to fulfill the ideal of the "perfect mother." When you are tired, frustrated, or confused, we want to give you permission to give yourself a break. As you and your partner become accustomed to parenting, a new routine will emerge and you'll feel your sense of panic, stress, and depression begin to lift. Remember your determination to breastfeed and stick with it as long as you can. You may feel that after a few weeks, breastfeeding was the best decision you ever made. Experiencing postpartum depression doesn't mean that you have to give up breastfeeding.

If, however, you are having a lot of trouble breastfeeding or feel that the demands of the breastfeeding life create too much stress for you and your new family, give yourself a window of time to make sure you really want to discontinue nursing. Remember that once you stop, it can be difficult to begin nursing again if you change your mind and want to keep nursing. If you *do* decide to stop nursing, well, we've said it before: *Don't feel guilty!* The health benefits you've given your child through breastfeeding, even for a short time, will remain with him throughout his lifespan—and that's something to be proud of.

If you are experiencing a deep postpartum depression that seems overwhelming to you or just won't lift no matter how hard you try, discuss your feelings with your physician as soon as you can. Postpartum depression is treatable with medication; getting help with it will only relieve the buildup of stress and anxiety that can accompany intense postpartum feelings.

Stress Management Techniques That Really Make a Difference

Stress is an unavoidable part of life, but managing it is a skill everyone can cultivate. Practice the following stress management basics, and encourage your family to practice them, too. Everyone will be happier, more relaxed, and healthier, because a tranquil and optimistic mental state facilitates a more resilient body with an enhanced capability for self-healing. All of these stress management techniques are directly beneficial to breastfeeding and holistic living.

MASSAGE

Everybody wants one, nobody wants to give one. All right, some people do like to give massages, and give them well, but these people are in short supply. The trick to getting a good massage is twofold: learn how to give a good massage, and then teach your partner how to do it. Take turns practicing to refine your skills. If you trade off nights, you won't have to get up and give a massage after the wonderful relaxation you have attained from receiving one. On the other hand, taking turns touching each other in this intimate way may bring other things to mind besides sleep. (You may want to agree ahead of time whether you will be engaging in a relaxing massage or a sensual massage—the former leads to sleep, and the latter . . . doesn't.)

Massage Basics for Adults

According to Tiffany Field, Ph.D., of the Touch Research Institute of the University of Miami School of Medicine, massage has been shown to increase mental alertness; alleviate stress, anxiety, and depression; boost immune system effectiveness; and reduce insomnia. The breastfeeding mother and her spouse or partner could use a little of each! Here are a few massage basics to get you more comfortable with the process. In general, massage strokes should move toward the heart.

Have your partner lie on his or her stomach on a relatively firm surface. Your bed is too soft for a really good massage, but a blanket on the floor is perfect. The recipient should expose as much skin as possible. (Nudity is nice, but not always appropriate.)

If you decide to use massage oil (a light vegetable or nut oil works, too—try sesame oil), put about a tablespoonful in your palms. Rub your hands together briskly to generate a little heat. (Be sure to use a blanket that can withstand a few oil stains, if you use oil.) Starting in the small of the back, gently but firmly rub your hands up both sides of the spine in long, smooth strokes, then down the sides of the back. Cover as much skin as you can with your hands, moving up and down in this pattern for several minutes with a long, firm stroking movement.

Walk your fingers up either side of the spine (do not press

No Time for a Massage?

If you think you don't have time to get a massage, let alone give one, think again. Here are some easy ways to sneak in a massage during the day.

⊚ When that dreaded alarm goes off in the morning, instead of groaning and hitting the snooze button, roll over and give your partner a "quickie" (a quickie *massage*). Tomorrow, ask him to do the same. You will find this more energizing than those ten extra minutes of half-sleep.

⊚ Give yourself a massage while you are showering. As you soap each part of your body, concentrate on deep, muscle-kneading strokes. A brisk facial massage while washing your face feels great, too. Invest in a soft face brush for a luxurious change in your routine.

⊚ Eat a quick, fresh salad for lunch, then swap shoulder rubs with a colleague at work (not on company time, of course) or an older child at home. Or, if no one else is to be found, relax, close your eyes, and rub your own shoulders, one at a time. Really work those muscles.

⊚ While dinner is cooking, tell your partner to sit back and relax. Give him a rejuvenating two-minute scalp massage, then ask him to return the favor after the meal is finished and the dishes are done. (You may want to agree that whoever does the dishes also gets the massage!)

⊚ According to those versed in the techniques of acupressure, a face massage can be sexually stimulating for women. Tell your partner this, then ask for a gentle face massage. Close your eyes and let yourself enjoy it utterly. Who knows where it will lead?

◎ Kids love to play with hair. Ask your older child to brush your hair and, if your hair is long enough, braid it. This feels wonderful. Then return the favor.

◎ After the baby goes to sleep, relax with your partner and take turns telling each other about your day. Whoever is talking gives a shoulder and back rub, or a foot and hand rub. Be sure to allow equal time (ten or fifteen minutes each). If one of you doesn't think you have anything to talk about, talk about your hopes for the future. And you can always talk about the baby. ("Today Junior bit the tips off three crayons and decorated the kitchen with spaghetti sauce!")

◎ Just before bed, take a bubble bath. When you are good and soapy, ask your partner for a soft, slow shoulder rub.

directly on the spine), pressing firmly. Walk them back down. Stroke down both buttocks with your hands, then back up. Stroke down each leg with a firm, flat hand. When you reach the foot, rub with firm strokes toward the toes, then pull gently on each toe. Stroke back up each leg, then massage the buttocks and lower back with firm, circular strokes.

Continue the circular strokes up each side of the back, concentrating on the areas all around the shoulder blades, the shoulder muscles, and the base of the neck.

Change your stroke to a firm, kneading motion, reaching deep into the muscles with your fingers as if you are picking up each muscle, squeezing it, and releasing it. (Be sure to tell your partner to speak up if you are massaging too hard.) Work around the shoulder blades again, then concentrate on the neck and shoulder area.

Thoroughly massage the scalp with your fingers. Have your partner turn over. Starting at the feet, rub each foot again firmly, then stroke up each leg with a flat hand. One at a time, take each hand and knead the palm, then rub down each finger and pull it gently. Stroke firmly up each arm. Stroke the shoulders, upper chest, stomach, then back up to the neck. Gently move your fingers in a circular motion along the hairline and over the forehead.

Very gently brush your fingers around the eye sockets, down the nose, and over the ears. Massage over each cheekbone, and rub each ear. Be careful during this part of the massage. Some people are very sensitive about having their face touched, but a facial massage can be extremely pleasant and relaxing.

Move back to the scalp, then grasp sections of hair and pull gently. End by raking your fingers lightly through the hair to the base of the neck and, with gentle, flat hands, sweeping down the back, the arms, the legs, and up the back again.

Infant Massage Basics

Infant massage is a great way to relax your baby and give her the benefit of your touch, which shouldn't, of course, be limited only to breastfeeding sessions. Even before a baby can see very well, her skin and sense of touch are ultrasensitive, so massage is an excellent way to communicate. Many colicky babies respond well to massage, but why limit your massages to when she is feeling terrible? Massage can be great at any time, and will make your baby more relaxed and happy (although if your baby doesn't seem to like it, stop—you can try again in a few days or weeks when she is in a more receptive mood).

Even babies who are only a few days old can benefit from a gentle massage. A recent study from the Touch Research Institute at the University of Miami School of Medicine reports that premature babies who received brief massages three times a day for ten consecutive days gained nearly 50 percent more weight and left the hospital an average of six days earlier than premature babies who didn't receive massage. Eight months later, the massaged babies still weighed more and were more advanced, both in mental and motor development.

Just as there are multiple massage techniques for grown-ups, you can find lots of different methods for massaging an infant. Here's one method to try. If you've just fed your baby, wait until she has had time to digest her meal to begin the massage; massaging a baby who just ate can trigger spitting up.

Lay your baby on your outstretched legs or on a comfortable towel or blanket on the floor, face up. Put a little baby lotion, cornstarch, or oil (*not* baby oil, which can clog pores—use vegetable or nut oil instead) in your palm and rub your hands together to warm them.

Slowly stroke your hands down each of the baby's legs, gently squeezing her thighs and moving down the legs to the feet with a "milking" motion. Gently rotate each ankle and massage each foot, gently pulling on each toe.

Next, massage each arm in a similar fashion, starting at the shoulder and gently squeezing and stroking down to the hand. Gently massage each hand and fingers.

Rub the baby's stomach and chest with wide, circular motions.

Turn the baby onto her stomach and use the same wide, circular motions on her back, then run your hands down her arms and legs again.

Gently place your hand on her forehead and lightly stroke from her forehead back to the nape of her neck several times.

Using your fingertips, gently massage your baby's shoulders and neck. Be very careful not to press on her spine.

Remove the baby's diaper and briefly massage her bottom. Replace the diaper.

Turn her back over again onto her back, and very gently brush your fingertips over her face and along her hairline. Gently stroke her head a few more times.

FATHER ALERT!

YOUR BIG CHANCE FOR INTIMACY!

True, you can't nurse your baby, but learning and practicing infant massage gives you a wonderful opportunity to establish an intimate physical bond. "Mom massages" will be welcome, too. Help your entire family to get into the massage habit, and you will all be happier and more relaxed.

Wipe off any excess oil or lotion with a towel when you are finished.

Your baby may or may not like any one of these steps. Experiment and do what feels natural, to better personalize the infant massage. Your baby is an individual, after all.

DEEP BREATHING RELAXATION TECHNIQUES

Whenever you feel overwhelmed by stress, take a quick, deep breathing break to restore your mental focus and calm and center your body. Deep breathing techniques take a little practice, but once mastered, are more beneficial than shallow "chest" breathing. When you breathe fully and deeply, rich oxygen is pumped through your bloodstream, nourishing and replenishing muscles and cells throughout your body. And more oxygen is pumped to your brain, allowing you to think more clearly and efficiently. Oxygen is one of your body's most important and frequently taken-for-granted "foods," making you stronger, healthier, and more vibrant.

For just ten or fifteen minutes, hand the baby over to Dad, an older sibling, or a helpful friend or relative. Go to your favorite

BREATHING VARIATIONS

The following variations can be incorporated into your deep breathing routines.

◎ Hold your breath for five or ten seconds between inhalation and exhalation.

◎ Gently hold one nostril closed with your finger and breathe in through the other nostril. Then switch nostrils to exhale. Repeat five times, then switch the inhaling and exhaling nostril. This is extremely relaxing and centering.

◎ Instead of exhaling with a "sss," exhale with a "hoo."

◎ Breathe lying on the floor with your knees bent at a ninety-degree angle and your feet resting on a chair. This helps pump more oxygen-rich blood faster to your brain.

room and shut the door, or settle into your favorite secluded spot outside. Sit comfortably with your back straight so your breathing isn't inhibited. (Don't lie down or you may fall asleep before you have the chance to relax completely and consciously.) Close your eyes. Very slowly, to the count of ten, breathe in through your nose, then even more slowly, to the count of twenty, breathe out through your mouth while making a "sss" sound. Do this ten times.

When you breathe in, put your hand on your lower abdomen. Rather than expanding your upper chest as you inhale, concentrate on expanding and lowering your diaphragm, a thick muscle at the base of your chest, just above your abdominal cavity. This movement allows for better lung expansion. Imagine your torso is a balloon. Fill it up from the bottom, starting by

expanding the abdomen. Your upper chest should be the very last
to fill with air. *Do not move your shoulders* at all when inhaling.
As you inhale, imagine healthy, energizing oxygen suffusing your
entire body and calming your overactive mind. With every exhalation, imagine negative energy leaving your body.

Complete your deep breathing session with some muscle
relaxation. Lie flat on a comfortable surface, letting your arms
and legs fall to the sides, palms facing up and toes facing out. In
yoga, this is called the "corpse pose." Consciously begin to relax
your body by following the instructions in the sequence below.
You may want to have someone read it out loud to you in a slow,
soothing tone. Or tape record the paragraph and play it to yourself while you perform the motions.

> *Feel the tension and stress of the day flowing out of your
> feet through the ends of your toes. Release the stored ten-
> sion from your ankles, shins, and calves. Feel it flowing
> down your lower legs and away. Imagine stress flowing
> out of your knees and thighs and hips. Your entire lower
> body becomes loose, relaxed, light, and completely free.
> Imagine all the tension in the center of your body
> swirling through your chest, your stomach, and your
> back, then slowly coming together and concentrating in
> your torso. Imagine jettisoning it from your belly button.
> It flows out of you like a river and is gone. Now the ten-
> sion in your hands falls away. Release the stress from
> your wrists, your lower arms, your elbows, and your
> upper arms. Anxiety remains balled up in your shoulders
> and neck. Feel it gathering around your top vertebrae,
> then splitting and shooting down each arm and out the
> ends of your fingers. Now, the last bits of tension in your
> jaw, your cheeks, around your eyes, your forehead, and
> your scalp fall away, leaving you completely, utterly
> relaxed. Lie very quietly and savor the relaxed feeling. If
> your mind wanders to problems that make you worry,*

banish them and concentrate all your energy on the feel of your relaxed body. Don't think, just feel. As your body sinks into the floor, spreading down roots to merge with the earth, imagine your soul slowly rising off the floor, through the roof, into the sky, then floating high above the earth, far beyond any mundane worries. You are completely relaxed, weightless, and free. Feel your breath moving in and out of your body. Smile.

Lie quietly in silence for a few minutes. If you fall asleep after all this, good, you probably needed the catnap. You may, however, feel extremely energized after this short relaxation session, ready to tackle the rest of the day, and ready to resume your admittedly unfree but dearly valued role as mom (or dad, or sibling—anyone can benefit from this exercise). Be sure to get up very slowly and savor the relaxed feeling as long as possible.

MEDITATION, VISUALIZATION, AND PRAYER

These stress management techniques are good follow-ups to deep breathing exercises. Depending on your personality and proclivity, make space in your day to meditate, visualize, or pray.

Meditation

"Meditate? Why? I'll just be thinking of everything I'm not doing while I'm sitting around staring at the wall and my baby's crying." Meditating doesn't have to be a tedious, impossible task. And you may find that time spent on a mental break gives you the focus and energy you need to pack more activity into your busy day. Beginners at mediation will find three methods useful. One is to clear the mind, allowing thoughts to flow through easily like a river of words that you passively observe. If that's too hard, try concentrating on a *particular* issue to be solved. Third is a consciousness "wake-up call." Each method can be beneficial at different times. Sit upright in a chair or on the floor; be comfortable but maintain good posture—don't slump down or choose a position that gives little support to the body, especially the lower back.

Clearing the mind. The first method involves letting go of conscious attachment to your thoughts. Some people do this by concentrating on a visual point or repeating a sound, such as a mantra like "om." You can choose any word, however, as long as it invokes a feeling of peace and tranquillity. Try "love" or "peace." Or choose a visual point of reference, such as a candle flame, a tree, or a cherished object. Focus on your point of reference and whenever other thoughts start to creep in, as they inevitably will, refocus on your sound or object. At first, it will seem virtually impossible. With practice, it gets easier. The purpose is to train your mind to clear itself and not allow it to be overwhelmed by clutter. The result is a sense of calm and control. This technique is most helpful when your mind is racing, you can't concentrate, and you feel "scattered."

Solving a problem. Focus on a particular dilemma that is causing you stress. Allow emotions to pass through you and note them as a detached observer. This technique is also good for when you have a nagging problem, even if you aren't sure what it is. If you feel like something is bothering you, concentrate on your feeling of discomfort. Don't try to solve your problem. In fact, try consciously to keep your mind from working out logical solutions. Simply acknowledge how you are feeling. The result will often be that images or thoughts will come to you that will make the problem suddenly clear, and solutions will become unexpectedly obvious.

Mindfulness: the wake-up call. The third meditation technique is slightly different. It can and should be practiced as often as possible while going about your everyday life. The technique simply involves becoming consciously aware of what you are doing. Most people go through life on "automatic" most of the time. Sometimes this is more efficient. It is certainly easier. But as often as you can, force your mind to take notice. What are you doing? What physical sensations are you feeling? What emotional feelings do you have? Are your shoulders tense? Is your brow furrowed? Are you twisting your hair, biting your nails, slouching like Quasimodo, rushing around, feeling irritated, ignoring your family, obsessing about your family? Are you cleaning, cooking, working, writing, resting, watching TV, exercising, eating? How does it feel to be you at this moment? The point is to reactivate your consciousness, to really *live* while you are merely existing, and to put stressful times in perspective. Thinking this way can truly heighten your experiences, and thinking this way while breastfeeding will increase your pleasure and deepen your memories about this cherished time in your life.

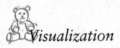

Visualization

Visualization is like meditation mixed with a good dose of imagination. It is great for helping you make decisions, attain goals, and solve problems. Begin by relaxing, closing your eyes, and breathing deeply, as for meditation, but then, instead of clearing your mind, push it into high gear. If you are feeling stressed, imagine yourself lying under a warm sun on a white beach. Imagine the feel of the warmth on your skin, the sand under you. Imagine the sound of the waves lapping gently on the shore. Or imagine yourself sitting quietly in a deep, calm, beautiful forest by a rippling stream. Or imagine yourself curled up beside a crackling fire as huge silver snowflakes drift down outside the window.

Now that you are calmer, visualize making the decision or confronting the problem that is bothering you. Concentrate on how you feel about the scenario you are visualizing. Then try it a different way, then a different way (all in your mind). By paying attention to how you feel as you visualize different solutions, you will become more attuned to which solution is the right one. Your creative mind may very well present you with solutions you hadn't considered before, or seemingly miraculous resolutions to situations you thought unsolvable.

If you've been having trouble breastfeeding, for example, every day for ten or fifteen minutes imagine yourself in an ideal location, wherever you feel calm and safe. Your beach, forest, or fireside spot would all be good choices. It needn't be a real place. Then imagine yourself holding your baby close to your heart. Imagine breastfeeding her. Feel how easy it is. Imagine her contented face. Feel the milk flowing. (You may actually experience the milk ejection reflex. As we said before, the mind is a powerful motivator!) Then, maintaining that calm, relaxed, loving feeling, take your baby into your arms and try again.

 Prayer

Not everyone believes in the power of prayer, but if you do, or if you are open to the idea, it is certainly worth a try. If you are religious, you probably have a good focus for prayer. If you are not, or haven't been for a long time, pray to the force of love in the universe, which is, in many religions, what God is.

Studies have demonstrated that prayer can be an effective aid to healing. In fact, a much-publicized 1982–1983 study showed that among patients in the Coronary Care Unit at San Francisco General Medical Center, those who were being prayed *for* by people they didn't know fared significantly better than those in a control group. Many other studies (some more scientifically rigorous than others, but all interesting) have shown that people who pray are generally happier and live longer. If you already pray, you probably aren't surprised. If you don't, why not give it a try?

When you pray, a few guidelines will help you focus. First, construct your thoughts in positive terms. The thoughts you send out into the universe should contain no negativism. Instead of

"Don't let my baby get sick" or "Stop me from feeling so depressed" or "Don't let us go bankrupt," rephrase your thoughts in positive terms: "Bless my baby with health and long life," "Fill my heart with joy and love," or "Provide us with what we need." Positive prayers are clearer, not clouded with doubt, fear, anxiety, and despair. Second, don't just ask for things. Reflect on love. Let yourself feel joy. Be thankful for all the good things you have. Send up praise to God, or whatever you feel directs the world toward goodness. Even if you are a skeptic and feel that life is random and not run by any higher force, the effect of consciously forming positive thoughts toward the world and your fellow humans might surprise you. To a large extent, the way you think shapes who you are.

THE POWER OF COMMUNICATION

Sometimes, all you need is someone to talk to. Not therapy, necessarily. Just a friend, your partner, a sibling, or a parent to listen without offering advice and without trying to solve your problems. Call it venting, call it peer counseling, call it a heart-to-heart. Whatever you call it, talking about your problems can sometimes be the most effective way to sort them out and see them objectively.

In addition, every breastfeeding mother should have at least one other mom she can call when things get rough. A network of moms with children of similar ages is even better. A weekly gathering of moms with their babies is ideal. Motherhood can be isolating, and if this is your first baby, no matter how much you read on the subject, sometimes problems or situations will arise that you can't find in any book. Enter the mom network! Talking out problems, sharing information, exchanging stories, and offering mutual, sympathetic support with and to new moms can make a potentially stressful time into a nurturing, growth-oriented time. If you don't have friends or siblings with kids, ask your pediatrician about other moms who attend his or her practice. Moms may already be meeting in a group you can join. Or start your own group. Post signs at your local library, talk to other moms in the park, or, if your city has a local parenting newsletter or magazine (many cities do), run an ad. Many, many, many other mothers out there feel just as you do. Finding them may just save your sanity.

But do more than just talk and network with others. Examine the words you use when *you* talk, your tone, your body language. What message are you *really* sending when you communicate with others? Some people tend naturally to be more positive than others. If you are a positive person, you are lucky. If you tend to see the glass as half empty, however, make an effort to notice when you are being negative, then consciously try to reverse your thinking. Instead of "This house will never be clean again!" think "I'll just keep the kitchen and bathroom clean for now. The rest isn't as important as my baby." Instead of "I can't stand the thought of one more person asking me to do something for them," think "I deserve some solitude tonight." Don't assume the worst and try not to see the bad side first. Positive thinking often can't change an actual situation, but it can change your attitude, your approach, and your reaction. But aren't those the essence of any situation? A positive approach minimizes stress and often precipitates solutions that a frantic, negative mind wouldn't see.

EXERCISE

We have been focusing largely on the mind and its significant effect on your body. Your body can also have a significant effect on your mind. Bodies were designed to move, to work, and to use their muscles. Neglecting your physical state can make you more vulnerable to the negative effects of stress.

When you were nine months pregnant, you probably couldn't have run a marathon. Now, however, your "excuse" is wailing in his playpen, wishing you would take him for a walk in the fresh air. So get moving! You'll look better, feel better, and be better. If anything in this world is a cure-all, it's exercise. Why should you make it a part of the breastfeeding life, you ask? Consider these reasons:

◎ Exercise is the *only* way to get those stretched and sagging tummy muscles back to their original shape. Time alone will not do the trick.

◎ Exercise alleviates depression, malaise, and fatigue.

◎ Exercise improves your circulation, which in turn alleviates swelling, leg cramps, pinched nerves, and a host of other complaints.

◎ Exercise increases your sex drive and an in-shape body will be more responsive.

◎ Exercise will help your muscles, joints, and organs return to their prepregnancy state more quickly.

◎ Exercise burns calories so you can eat more and stay healthier.

◎ Exercise makes you feel great about yourself.

◎ Exercise gives you incredible energy and makes your brain work more efficiently.

◎ Exercise doesn't need to be intense, painful, or unpleasant. A brisk walk in the sunshine, a few sit-ups and knee push-ups while watching TV, and dancing to your favorite music all count as exercise. The trick is to do it almost every day.

◎ Exercise helps you live longer. It's a documented fact!

After the rigors of childbirth, your body will need to recover. For the first six weeks or so, don't worry too much about getting a lot of exercise. Your body is working on repairing itself and your milk supply is getting established. If you are restless and feel an intense need to get moving, take that daily walk in the fresh air with your little one. Don't jump right back into what you were doing before at the same level. Let your body heal.

After the six-week period, gradually resume the exercise program you followed before you got pregnant. If you were sedentary, this is a good time to start an exercise program. Talk to your doctor to come up with an exercise program that works for your fitness level and general state of health. The most important thing is to listen to your body. If you feel pain, dizziness, or any other discomfort, slow down. If you feel great, gradually increase your activity. Lochia, the fluid similar to menstrual blood which you pass for several weeks after childbirth, and which gradually lightens in color and decreases in flow, should not change to bright red after exercising. If it does, you are going too fast. If you overdo it and experience bleeding or other worrisome physical symptoms such as fainting or pain, call your doctor right away.

Your exercise plan should include three facets:

◎ *An aerobic workout, such as aerobic dancing, jogging, or brisk walking, which increases your heart rate.*

◎ *Strength training, such as weight lifting, push-ups and sit-ups, even carrying a baby around all day, which builds your muscles.*

◎ *Stretching, which lengthens your muscles and makes you more flexible.*

Don't forget to warm up and warm down for at least five minutes before and after any vigorous exercise, to protect your body against injury.

Exercise classes of all types abound, and taking a class can have multiple benefits. It gets you out of the house, gives you some time to yourself (many health clubs now include free child care), introduces you to new friends, and instructs you on the

ACHING BACK? WORK THAT TUMMY!

Now that your belly is quickly flattening and your swayback is straightening out, why is your back still so sore? Not only is your entire skeleton adjusting and realigning after pregnancy, but you've been walking around carrying a baby all day. Your back isn't used to this new adjustment of weight, and muscle strain is the common result. The solution? A strong abdomen. The stronger your stomach muscles, the better they will be able to support your back. Get in the habit of doing a few sit-ups every night, adding a few each week. Take it slow, though. You're not in the Olympics! Just do what you can comfortably achieve. Your back will thank you, and you'll fit back into those jeans even faster.

proper methods for whatever sport interests you. Use the following chart to help you determine what type of exercise you might enjoy the most, according to your personality type. If you don't see yourself described, survey the various activities. Something may spark your interest.

Any exercise that appeals to you is worth a try. Use your imagination. Experiment. Most of all, get up off that couch and get moving. Children with couch potato parents are much more likely to be couch potato kids. If your baby sees you being active, she'll be more likely to be an active child and a healthier adult.

Extremely strenuous exercise, however, may not be a good idea when you are breastfeeding if it causes you to lose weight too quickly or puts too much of a stress on your system. Also, certain high-risk or high-speed sports, such as hang gliding, sky diving, downhill skiing, rock climbing, even ice skating and rollerblading, pose certain physical risks that are best avoided. Your baby needs you, intimately and constantly, while nursing

IF YOU ARE . . .	THEN YOU MIGHT ENJOY . . .
musical, artistic, creative	dance classes, such as ballet, jazz, ballroom dancing, or Latin dancing aerobics, such as Jazzercise exercise classes for moms and babies (any mom might enjoy these)
flexible, spiritual, interested in other cultures	yoga tai chi martial arts
athletic, social, strong	team sport leagues such as volleyball, tennis, basketball, racquetball, or soccer health club memberships weight lifting
quiet, private, good at concentrating	running bicycling (on a real bike or a stationary bike) indoor pool swimming
a nature lover, would rather do anything outdoors	hiking gardening

IF YOU ARE . . .	THEN YOU MIGHT ENJOY . . .
	swimming outdoors
	cross-country skiing
	sailing
	canoeing or kayaking (keep it safe)
completely and totally unathletic, repulsed by anything resembling exercise, easily bored	long walks in the park or the country
	going out dancing with friends
	playing with children
	renting a variety of exercise videos, so you don't get tired of the same ones
	riding a stationary bike or walking on a treadmill with a rack for a book, or while watching TV

(and beyond). An injury or worse could be tragic not only for you but for this new life you have just brought so carefully into the world. Be careful and sensible. You'll have plenty of time for risk-taking after the important business of parenting a young child is past.

WHEN WILL MY LIFE BE MY OWN AGAIN?

Another common cause of stress in new mothers is something many mothers don't want to admit: although you love your family and are devoted to your baby, sometimes you have fantasies of running away, disappearing to a place where nobody *needs* you. It's true that you are profoundly needed these days, and although that can be rewarding, it can also be draining. Your baby is constantly nursing and you may resent not being able to do all the things you enjoy, like having a couple glasses of wine, taking a vacation, wearing a bikini, making love in the middle of the day, drinking nothing but diet soda all day long. Sometimes you really miss your past life, the you who was free and unencumbered, full of potential, ambitious, popular, sexy. Now you feel like a milk factory, or an automaton programmed for routine baby care and household drudgery. You might feel like you are spread so thin between motherhood, work, and your marriage that you have become transparent.

The only way to avoid burnout is to make sure your own needs are met. A baby can't be expected to know you have needs, too, although this is an important concept he will have to learn eventually. Dad and other kids, however, may need to be reminded once in a while. Don't fool yourself into thinking you shouldn't have to remind them. People tend to take the path of least resistance, and if that means letting you do everything, you may find yourself suffering from Super Mom syndrome, with a stress level to match. It isn't worth it. If you need some time alone to sit outside in the sun, put on headphones and listen to your favorite music, read a novel or newspaper, or just plain regroup, take it.

If you feel guilty about meeting your own needs, perhaps at the expense of other family members, think of it this way: if your needs are met, you will be happier, calmer, more efficient, more loving, and a much better mother and partner. Everyone will win.

TWENTY WAYS TO SNEAK EXERCISE INTO YOUR DAY

Yes, you have time to exercise, especially since the more you exercise, the more energy you'll have to accomplish every-thing faster and more efficiently. You'll find that the more you keep active in little ways throughout the day, the faster you will lose those pregnancy pounds. Sure, breastfeeding helps, by burning calories without exercise—but it doesn't do much for your muscle tone, so incorporate more move-ment into your day using the following strategies.

◎ When the alarm first goes off, before you get out of bed, stretch from head to toe, circle each foot and each hand a few times in each direction, then squeeze your buttocks muscles together twenty times.

◎ Get up thirty minutes before the baby usually wakes up and do an exercise video or exercise program on TV (many such programs are on in the morning—check sports channels and public television).

◎ When playing with your baby, lie on your back with him on your stomach, and do as many sit-ups as you can.

◎ Do upside-down push-ups. Lie on your back, hold the baby in both hands facing you, and lift her up and down. Make it a game—babies love this, and it is great for your arm muscles, too.

◎ Put your baby in a stroller and go on a brisk walk. Really look around you and enjoy the sunshine, the trees, the flowers, or whatever scenery you have. Point things out to the baby as you go.

◎ If you're watching TV anyway, do crunches, push-ups, leg lifts, and jumping jacks until you are very tired (or until your family makes you stop because you are driving them crazy!).

◎ While standing over the stove waiting for water to boil, a sauce to thicken, or vegetables to cook, do as many buttocks squeezes as you can. Then raise and lower yourself on your toes as many times as you can—great for your calf muscles. Stretch after you are done, so your leg muscles don't cramp.

◎ Make homemade bread without the dough hook attachment to your mixer. Kneading bread dough is great for your arms.

◎ Vacuum the entire house as fast as you can. For added strength-training: if your baby isn't scared of the vacuum cleaner, pick her up and carry her around while you vacuum.

◎ Play "I'm coming to get you" with your toddler. Very exhausting. Then switch to a fast-paced game of "hide and seek."

◎ Let Dad watch the baby for thirty to sixty minutes, perhaps when he first gets home from work and the baby hasn't seen him for a while. Go for a nice, peaceful, solitary walk or run. The family dog might like to join you. He can probably use a break from the baby, too!

◎ Wash all the windows in your house, inside and out. Not only is this a great arm workout, but you will be uplifted by the sparkling view you forgot you had. If you still have energy left, wash all the mirrors, too.

◎ When you are feeling tense and the baby is screaming, put on some energetic music and dance. Your toddler will love to dance with you, either separately or in your arms. Your younger infant will love to watch you, and may think the sight is quite hilarious. Make him laugh!

⊚ Squeeze your buttocks muscles while standing in line at the supermarket, while waiting at a red light, while talking on the phone, and whenever else you are just "wasting time" getting something done without moving. This is a good time to do Kegel exercises, too, which aren't just for pregnant women. They'll help your body get back in shape, and can improve your sex life. (Kegel exercises involve squeezing and releasing the muscles you would use to stop a flow of urine. Yes, those muscles.)

⊚ If you have stairs in your house or outside your front or back door, whenever you are about to climb up them, stop and put your toes on the edge of the first stair. Lift and lower yourself ten to twenty times, then proceed up the stairs.

⊚ Feeling frustrated? Jog in place as hard and as fast as you can for thirty seconds. (Remember the *Flashdance* workout? Just like that. A great tension reliever.)

⊚ Before you go to bed each night, spend ten minutes stretching. Roll your head gently forward and from side to side (not back). Lift your arms high over your head and reach, then reach to the left and right. Slowly drop your arms down and bend over to touch your toes (or as close as you can get). If you need more guidance, hundreds of books and videos offer a variety of stretching and flexibility routines. A short yoga workout is a good relaxer, too.

⊚ Give your partner a really intense massage. Use your muscles. (But don't hurt him!)

⊚ Have sex. Make it *workout* sex. (Enough said.)

⊚ When you are feeling clumsy, fat, or lazy, take a five-minute break. Sit down. Close your eyes. Take a few deep breaths. Visualize yourself fit, strong, and healthy. Imagine yourself successfully engaging in your favorite sport.

Watch your muscles work. See how great you look. Feel the endorphin rush. Believe in your physical abilities. This isn't actual, physical exercise, of course, but it will help to get you there. You can do it

Plus, once again, you will be setting an example for your baby, who will see that mothers aren't switchboards, through which everything should be channeled, or servants, hired to meet everyone's needs, or deities, able to be everywhere, do everything, and know all.

So, what are your needs? You may not even remember! Pull out a pen and paper and make a list. What *do* you need and what things do you love to do that you just can't find the time for now? Ask your spouse or partner to make a similar list. Then, discuss your lists together and try to come up with some creative ways to enjoy your favorite activities. You may find that embracing family life doesn't have to mean giving up your identity. Do your best to enjoy this new life passage of parenthood, to incorporate it into who you are.

Stressed out about breastfeeding? Relax! Focus on the stress management techniques you've learned in this chapter and concentrate on taking each precious moment of life as it comes. Feel good about what you are doing for your baby by choosing to try breastfeeding, and never lose sight of the miracle of life you are witnessing as your baby grows strong and healthy. That'll put most stressful events right into perspective.

8

BREASTFEEDING, YOUR RELATIONSHIP, AND LOVING THE NEW YOU

WELCOME TO PARENTHOOD

DAD didn't used to be "Dad"; he was your friend, your lover, your life-partner. And you . . . ? Well, now when you look in the mirror, you see this vaguely familiar person everyone is calling "Mom." The human milk factory. Wow. What happened? How could such a tiny little baby cause such a profound change in your lives, and in your ideas about yourselves? Your little one is putting your relationship through some growing pains. The first step in productively maintaining and improving your relationship is to know, specifically, how it has changed—and how it is growing. Identify the changes, then get to work on nurturing a new level of support, love, affection, and yes, even passion with the man in your life.

SEX AND BREASTFEEDING

No, not sex! That's what got you *into* this mess! Yes, but aren't you glad it did? In our culture, of course, sex is more than just babymaking. It is an important aspect of a marriage or committed relationship, perhaps more so to your partner than to you (although this isn't always the case, by any means), and *especially now*. You may wonder why sex is so important now, when you may feel so much like not having it. It is important because you need to reestablish physical contact with your partner. The breastfeeding life is not a celibate life! Your partner's hormones are just the way they have always been. For many men (again, there are always exceptions, of course), a good sexual relationship with his partner is crucial to communication and closeness. "Dad" is your partner in more than parenthood; let him help you reawaken your sexual side. (Some women do not experience a decreased sex drive after childbirth, which is also normal.)

Right now, your hormones are at work, focused on milk production and maternal instincts, not on reproduction. Your estrogen levels are low, which can suppress your sex drive and make sex uncomfortable (due to dryness). Your body is telling you it isn't ready to make more babies yet. You should listen to your body: that's what birth control is for. Use it until you are quite sure, mentally and physically, that you are ready for another pregnancy, because you may not be able to recognize accurately when you start ovulating again.

Until you start ovulating, sexual feelings may not arise on their own. You may need a little extra motivation. Sex is largely a matter of the mind, so believe in your ability to become reacquainted with your sexual side and it will happen, sooner or later. The important thing is to let your partner help you rather than shutting him out.

For the first six weeks or so, your body is healing from childbirth and your baby's needs require your primary attention. After that, you can remind your body of pleasures apart from motherhood. You may feel resistant to the idea because you are so focused on parenting and nursing your child. Focus is good, but you and your baby don't exist in a vacuum. You are part of a family, and you need to fight the urge to ignore everything beyond the baby and you. You are experiencing a good and productive natural instinct designed to keep a baby nourished and protected at all costs, and you should relish it, but you cannot let it consume you. You are a mother, but you are more: you are a friend, a lover, and a partner. Remember?

That being said, know that it is perfectly normal to feel completely uninterested in sex, to worry about the baby instead of concentrating on making love, to be self-conscious about milk leaking from your breasts when you do become aroused (though many men find this arousing), to feel that mothers aren't supposed to be sexy, to be too exhausted or "touched out" to want any kind of contact with your partner at all, and to be hesitant to discuss the issue. Have faith that these obstacles can be overcome. It just takes a little planning, and some persistence.

TEN WAYS TO GET IN THE MOOD

Now for the persistence part. The following ideas may help you get "in the mood" again. And remember, just because you aren't in the mood at first doesn't mean your mood won't change. As we've said before, the mind is an amazing thing. Just as smiling can make you feel happy, sexy behavior can make you feel sexy. Most importantly, talk to your mate. Let him know your unsexy feelings have nothing to do with *him*, and ask him to help you find them again.

While breastfeeding, you may feel—at least at first—that your breasts just aren't ready to do double duty for both your partner and your baby. If your breasts are too sensitive from breastfeeding, or you feel you'd like your partner to focus on other areas during romantic encounters, discuss it with him. Simply having him hold your breasts gently may be a warm and comforting way for you both to feel intimate and connected. Try not to take your breasts completely "off limits." By accepting and exploring the physical changes in your body together, you may become closer than you ever thought possible.

FATHER ALERT!

ROMANCING A MOM

Dad, you have been a saint. You may have abstained from having sex with your partner in the last month or so of pregnancy because it was too awkward or uncomfortable for her. Then the doctor said to wait six weeks after the birth of your baby. Now the six weeks are up and you are wondering when you're going to get the green light. But whenever you are alone together, the baby cries, the baby needs to nurse, your partner falls asleep, or she just doesn't seem interested. You can read the signals. No one wants to approach someone who doesn't want to be approached. Understand that her hormones are making things difficult. They are telling her it is too soon to make another baby. They don't know about the miracle of birth control.

A large part of helping your partner get reoriented to making love is in the setup. Get in the habit of touching her in affectionate but nonsexual ways. Set a romantic scene, with candles, sparkling cider, a light supper you have prepared. Offer to give her a massage or a foot rub. Brush her hair. Continually remind her that she's beautiful and show her that she's sexy to you. If she can get used to touching again without thinking it will necessarily or immediately lead to sex, she may be more open to the idea. Then, of course, the more she is touched, the more she will realize she *does* want to have sex again.

And don't be surprised if you've got a new take yourself on the whole sex thing now that you're a father. The sexual union between you and your partner has a new richness and meaning now that it has produced a child. And it can produce another one! Allow this to deepen the level of intimacy and sharing you experience with your partner. If it scares you, talk with her about it. Most likely, she's feeling the same fear, exhilaration, and wonder about it all.

Here we go, ten ways to get in the mood:

Clean Up Your Act. Nothing will make you feel *less* sexy than realizing you haven't showered in three days and your clothes are covered with baby spit-up. Try to take a shower or a bath every day. Don't worry about primping, but get really clean, brush back or tie back your hair, and put on clean clothes. No clean clothes to be found? Delegate laundry duty. Feeling clean and refreshed will make you feel more desirable, even if you still feel overweight or flabby. Try taking a shower or bath just after the baby has gone to bed, then approach your husband when your hair is still wet, wearing just a towel. Tell him you need him to put lotion on your back. Who says you need to be at the beach?

Get and Give a Sensual Massage. The sensual massage differs from the regular massage, which circumvents the sexual areas of the body. When giving a sensual massage, don't concentrate on the erogenous zones at first, but don't avoid them, either. Use lots of scented massage oil, and after the body is relaxed, rub the ears, the face, the chest, the genitals, all lightly, even teasingly. Show your partner how to do this, too. Don't give in right away to your urge to stop the massage and start making love. Draw out the massage until you and your partner are very aroused. Delayed gratification can be even *more* gratifying.

Have a Light Supper. Nothing makes you feel more sluggish and unattractive than a huge, heavy meal. Instead of stuffing yourself, serve a light salad with bread for dinner, and have some fresh fruit for dessert. Eat by candlelight and play classical music or soft jazz. After dinner, ask your husband to slow dance.

Send Him Flowers at the Office. Why not? He'll be touched that you are thinking of him that way, and he'll know something's up. Depending on how daring you are (or how nosy his co-workers are), write something more or less racy on the card. After the baby is in bed, surprise your partner with a flowing, silky, sexy-but-comfortable nightgown or negligee (make sure it is something that makes *you* feel sexy).

Ask Him to Wash Your Feet. Have a large bowl, perfumed soap, lotion, and a soft sponge in a convenient location. Point him in the right direction, then sit back and really enjoy it. *Don't* feel guilty about relaxing with total abandon.

Take a Deep Breath, Hire a Trusted Baby-sitter, and Go on a Date. Nothing will make you feel more like your old self again than a good-old-days date. You may find it difficult to leave your baby, especially the first time, but everyone will benefit if you indulge in "couple time" every so often. Have dinner at a nice restaurant (but eat lightly). See a movie. Hold hands in the theater. Go for a walk through the city or a local park during the afternoon, or take a moonlit stroll after dark. Go to a carnival, indulge at an ice cream parlor, or meet in a coffee shop for cappuccino (decaf is best!). Go to the country and pick wildflowers. Stroll through the zoo holding hands. Have a picnic. Try not to talk about the baby. All right, just don't talk *only* about the baby. If you're at a loss about what else to talk about, try some of the following questions:

◎ *I think your best quality is . . . (You fill in the blank—be specific and detailed.) What do you think my best quality is?*

◎ *If you had a million dollars, what is the first thing you would do?*

◎ *If you could solve just one of the world's many challenges, which one would it be?*

◎ *Who do you consider your hero?*

◎ *Conduct a favorite inventory: favorite color, holiday, flower, article of clothing, cologne, place, hobby, song, movie, president, animal, food, dessert, drink, relative, sleeping position, state, etc. How many did you already know? Remember times when you've shared your favorite things.*

◎ *If you could have a vacation home anywhere in the world, where would it be?*

◎ *In what interesting location would you most like to make love?*

◎ *What's the one thing you would like to do while making love that you've never done? (Be prepared for anything . . . and don't ask if you don't want to know!)*

◎ *Wanna play strip poker? (If he says yes, do it—but you should probably wait until you get home.)*

Make Out Every Day for a Week. Sit on his lap, meet him at the door, catch him in the car. The rule is: no sex. Kiss, hug, fondle, enjoy touching. Keep this up for one week. By the end of the week, you should both be good and ready to make love. Pretend it is your first time. And, indeed, in some ways it is!

Get the Bedroom Really Clean. Remove magazines, clutter, baby toys. Fill the room with candles (lots and lots of candles, but not in positions where they could get knocked over or ruin any surfaces). Turn down the bed and place rose petals on the sheets for some romantic aromatherapy. Think *boudoir*. How can you help but feel sexy in a place like that? If your new family is experimenting with a family bed, don't despair! If you've got a guest room, turn your attention there. If not, try the sofa in the living room or target another area of the house and schedule a rendezvous; you can even consider getting a sitter and checking into a hotel for the evening—who says you have to stay the whole night? Room service!

Read Erotica. Different from pornography, erotica is sensuous writing meant to get you in the mood. Read it alone or, if you are feeling really uninhibited, read it out loud to your partner (or have him read it out loud to you). Try anything by Anaïs Nin. Try the *Kama Sutra*. Browse the bookstores. You can even find magazines with erotica. Alternatively, rent a romantic and/or erotic movie, such as any of the following (this list is a completely random sampling of romantic movies—some are steamier than others):

9½ Weeks	The Competition
An Affair to Remember	Cyrano de Bergerac
As Good As It Gets	Doctor Zhivago
Ball of Fire	The English Patient
Barefoot in the Park	Far and Away
Breakfast at Tiffany's	Four Weddings and a Funeral
Bridges of Madison County	Frankie and Johnny
Bull Durham	The French Lieutenant's Woman
Casablanca	Ghost

Gone With the Wind	Romancing the Stone
Henry & June	Romeo and Juliet
Holiday	A Room with a View
Indiscreet	Roxanne
Intermezzo	Sabrina
It Happened One Night	Say Anything
L.A. Story	Sense and Sensibility
Last Tango in Paris	Shadowlands
Magnificent Obsession	She's Having a Baby
Moonstruck	Sleepless in Seattle
Much Ado About Nothing	Titanic
Out of Africa	The Way We Were
Phenomenon	When Harry Met Sally
Pretty Woman	Working Girl

Tell Your Partner . . . Too often, couples don't *talk*. Here are a few things to take a deep breath and tell him.

◎ *I really like it when we're making love and you . . . (Fill in the blank—tell* him!*)*

◎ *Believe it or not, I would feel incredibly relaxed and sexy if some-one cleaned the entire house. (Hint, hint!)*

◎ *I think it's really sexy to see you being a good father to our baby.*

◎ *I love you! (Some couples just don't say it enough.)*

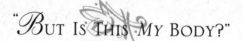

"BUT IS THIS MY BODY?"

Okay, we hear you. It's one thing to get in the mood for love, and it's quite another thing to face the physical truth that you're no longer that perky, prepregnancy you. Are those really your breasts? Didn't they used to have at least a degree of . . . buoyancy? And could that be your rear view? What about those veins, those stretch marks, that droopy stomach? How are you supposed to feel good about yourself, looking like *this*? Two ways. One, you don't look all that bad. People tend to obsess about the minutiae. Chances are, your newly acquired imperfections are far less noticeable than you think. Two, many of these imperfections will correct themselves with time. Those that don't you should wear like a medal. You are a mother now—be proud! So your body doesn't look like a teenager's anymore. So what? (If you are one of those few women whose body bounces right back to teenager quality three months after childbirth, keep it quiet—we don't want to hear about it!) You are a grown woman, and the fact that you have given birth and are a mother can be extraordinarily attractive and sexy.

If you are worried that your partner no longer finds your body appealing, talk to him. Explain that you are feeling a little insecure about your appearance. Tell him you need to know that he is still attracted to you. Why wait for him to come up with the reassuring words on his own? Chances are, he just assumes you know how he feels. There is nothing wrong with coaxing the information to the surface.

LOOKING (AND *FEELING*) GOOD AGAIN

During the first few months with your new baby, you probably won't give much thought to your appearance, until the real world starts to infringe upon you again. When you are ready to claim your fair share of vanity, begin with these easy steps. Nothing drastic, though—you may want to hold back a while on that urge for a tattoo!

◎ *Get a professional haircut. You don't need to go dramatically different, although many mothers decide to cut their long hair short. Even if you just get a trim, get dressed and go out for the professional treatment. It will make you feel pampered. However,* **don't make a major change right away when you may still be on the postpartum roller coaster.** *When you feel like yourself again, you may regret that shade of red that looked so good in the picture, or getting that buzz cut. Also, don't get a perm for at least three or four months. Your hair isn't back to normal yet and may not react well. And don't be alarmed when, a few months postpartum, your hair begins to fall out in bushels. You didn't lose the normal amount of hair during pregnancy, so you'll be losing it all at once afterward. You may even get a few near-bald spots, but don't despair—it will all grow back.*

◎ *Give yourself a facial. First, wash your face with a gentle soap. Heat water in a teakettle, then pour it into a large bowl. Drape a towel over your head and tent it over the bowl. Steam your face while breathing slowly and deeply for ten minutes. (Never steam your face over water boiling on the stove—that steam is too hot and could burn you.) After steaming, splash your face with warm water, then with a soft face brush or cloth, gently massage your face using small, circular motions. Rinse again with warm water. Apply a homemade mask (see the next page for recipes), place two chilled cucumber slices on your eyes (reduces puffiness), then lie back and relax for fif-*

teen minutes. Gently but thoroughly wash off the mask, then splash your face ten times with ice-cold water. Your complexion will glow!

Mask for oily skin: Mix one egg yolk, the juice of one-fourth of a lemon, and two tablespoons brown rice flour (or raw brown rice ground to a powder in a blender). Apply to face. (This makes enough for two masks, so share with a friend.)

Mask for dry skin: Mix two teaspoons cornstarch, one teaspoon honey, and a few drops of strong chamomile tea. Apply to face.

Mask for anyone: Mix one-half cup cooked oatmeal with one egg yolk and enough water to make a thick paste. This can also be used as a facial scrub.

◎ *Give your breasts a facial!* Sound strange? Not at all! Neck and chest skin show signs of aging just like your face, especially if they've been sun damaged. People in many cultures apply body packs to the sensitive neck and chest area to keep them youthful and refreshed. You've recently been through weight gain and loss, and your breasts have experienced their own radical changes. Give yourself a treat and try the following homemade recipes (both can also be used for the face):

Body pack I: Mix two blocks fresh, drained tofu with a little oat flour or rice flour (you can grind oats or raw rice in a blender to make the flour) to make a thick, creamy paste. Apply to neck, chest, and breasts (not to nipples) and leave on for fifteen minutes, then rinse off with cool water.

Body pack II: Apply whipped egg whites to your neck, chest, and breasts (not to nipples). Leave on for fifteen minutes, then rinse off with cool water. (A great way to use leftover egg whites!)

◎ *Revamp your wardrobe.* Pull everything out of your closet. Pack up all your maternity clothes and stash them away (or give them away if you don't plan on having a "next time"). See what's left. You probably don't even remember you had some of those clothes! Survey what you have and what you need. Throw away or give away anything that doesn't make you feel really good. Make a list *of the basic necessities you require, and the extras you would like. Go shopping. If you still don't fit into your old clothes, buy just a few things in your "in-between" size. You shouldn't have to wait until you lose all the weight to look well dressed. And buy some luxurious sleepwear while you're at it.*

◎ *If you haven't already, organize a regular exercise schedule (see chapter 7). Not only will exercise help you lose weight and allow you to eat more, but it will give your complexion a rosy glow, energize you, clear your mind, boost your mood, and generally improve your life. A brisk, thirty-minute walk five or six times a week plus muscle toning exercises like sit-ups and push-ups should do the trick, but consider the multitude of other options, too. Truly regular, moderately vigorous exercise is without question the best thing you can do to improve your appearance, health, and self-esteem.*

Don't be surprised if childbirth and breastfeeding have changed your feelings about your appearance. The breastfeeding life is so different from the preparenthood life that you will feel, in many ways, like a completely different person. Sure, there will be moments when you long for the old you, but having a baby is a maturing and empowering experience, and many women find that their appearance reflects that. You've created life. You are beautiful, and growing stronger every day.

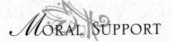

MORAL SUPPORT

Maybe even more than sex, you both need moral support. It is easy to feel like you do nothing but give, and to feel resentful that you aren't getting enough back. This kind of thinking is a trap. Your resentment will cut off support from others, not encourage

FATHER ALERT!

JOIN THE CLUB

Your partner knows you love her, and she knows you find her attractive. The profound physical changes she has experienced through pregnancy and childbirth, however, may have made her a little insecure about her appearance and her changing identity. Remember that right now she is pouring everything into your baby. It can be easy for a new mother to forget that she is a person on her own, and worthy of love just because she is who she is. Enter *you!* You can help her self-esteem reestablish itself with a few sincere words and actions that are *not* aimed at her mothering abilities (although she'll like to hear that you think she is a good mother, too).

Consider the following ideas for boosting self-esteem, then carry out the ones you think she'll appreciate. If you feel silly, do it anyway. If she resists your attempts to give her a boost, be persistent. Sooner or later, she'll believe you, and believe in herself. The more you give to her, the more she will be able to give back and the richer your relationship will be.

- Catch her from behind, wrap your arms around her, and whisper in her ear that she has never been as sexy to you as she is now.

- Mail her a card for no reason at all. Address it, "To my lover."

- Offer to wash her hair. Tell her how great she looks with her hair wet.

- Write a love poem to her and leave it where she can find it when you aren't home. (Not creative? Write out a famous love poem and dedicate it to her. Tell her it made you think of her.)

- Think of something she knows about that you don't know about (American history? cooking? car engines? Spanish? politics?). Ask her to teach you or explain it to you. Then *let* her. Really listen. Ask thoughtful questions.

- Give her a pedicure. Paint her toenails and blow them dry.

- Hold her hand in public.

- Bring her a single flower (be creative—find something other than red roses, unless she really loves them) every day for a week. By the weekend, she'll have a beautiful bouquet.

- Offer to take the baby for the afternoon, and urge her to spend some time doing whatever she wants to do, baby-free (even if she just stays home and relaxes in another room, in which case you must resist the temptation, no matter how strong, to bother her with questions).

it. To get, you need to give, but give in the right way. You need to spend time together—no easy trick with a screaming infant in the house—and you need to know how to listen.

The best thing you can do for your relationship *right now* is to make a commitment to spend at least thirty minutes of uninterrupted time together every single day, when the baby is napping or has gone to sleep for the night. *Every single day.* During this precious thirty minutes, you should unplug the phone and leave the television off. Talk. Don't consciously feel like you need to pour out moral support during this time. Simply talking will do the trick. If you start to argue, stop immediately and regroup. Tell each other that you can argue at any other time, but not during this thirty minutes. Stay positive. Talk about the good things that happened to you that day. If something is really bothering one of you, take turns "venting." The listener must listen with complete, nonjudgmental sympathy. Don't feel you have to give advice or solve any problems. Just listen, and you will be doing what your partner needs. Eventually you will come to depend on these thirty-minute sessions (or longer if you have the time) as a cornerstone of strength in your partnership. Without them, you may go for weeks or months without really talking, and this is dangerous for your relationship, let alone your self esteem.

You need each other, now more than ever. Don't spend your days wishing your partner was there for you. Take an active part in your commitment to each other. Consciously and with love, decide to be together physically and emotionally. An added bonus: your child will see how good unions are made, and will be better prepared to have one, too, someday.

WHAT ABOUT SINGLE MOMS?

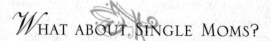

In 1993, the U.S. Census Bureau reported that single motherhood had increased sixty percent over the previous decade. That means that nearly one quarter of America's never-married women are deciding to become single mothers. If you've made the decision to have a child on your own, you'll still face many of the issues we've discussed in this chapter, such as embracing your role as a parent, reconnecting to your feelings of sexuality, and loving your new physical self. With a strong support group of friends and family, you'll find you and your baby nurtured by a loving network that will bolster your confidence and give you the emotional and physical help you'll need to balance the responsibilities of parenting solo. No ready network? Go out and build one; there are lots of single mothers out there. Contact Single Mothers by Choice or Parents Without Partners (see Resources). Be tenacious—and we know you are!

The choice to breastfeed your baby as a single mother requires a hefty amount of determination, perseverance, and logistical acumen—particularly if you're trying to support yourself and your baby financially at the same time. If possible (or

MONEY TALKS

If you are like many couples, money is the subject about which you argue more than any other. To make matters worse, finances may be strained now if you have taken significant time off work or if you have quit your job to stay home with the baby for a while. Dad may feel the added burden of bearing the family's complete financial responsibility alone. You may feel guilty about not doing your financial share, even if you know in your heart that staying home with your baby is more important to you. Even if you don't have a decreased income, your expenses are up. Diapers, visits to the pediatrician, diapers, baby clothes and supplies, diapers . . . why did you ever think you could afford this tiny little person?

If you and your partner have different approaches to money, the situation can be further aggravated. One of you may be a spender, the other a saver. Or, if you both tend to be extravagant, you may feel like no one is in control, and that can be extremely stressful. The best way to handle financial problems is to make a sensible budget and stick to it. Easier said than done, you say? True, but budgeting can give you confidence in and control over your financial situation and, like any good habit, the more you get used to doing it, the easier it becomes. Plus, if you have planned to stay home with the baby and the family will suddenly have a reduced income, a budget is crucial, first to see if quitting your job is actually feasible, and second, to help you get by on money you probably already thought wasn't quite enough.

When money becomes an issue, remember that being together as a family is more important than anything money can buy. And just remember how much money you're saving by breastfeeding your baby! That should cheer you both up.

desirable), consider moving in with a friend or relative for the first few months, at least. Or consider asking friends and family members to take shifts staying with you to help you take care of things. Explore flexible work schedules with your employer; a work-at-home arrangement is best, if possible.

As for dating and romance, why not? If it's something you want to do, go for it. Married, single, or divorced, motherhood is sexy!

9

❦ LIFE ON THE OUTSIDE

ℛEJOINING THE WORLD

OMETIME between your baby's sixth week and first birthday, the thought will occur to you: I'm going to have to get back out there. Not just out to the store, or the park, or around the block, but out there in the working, adult world. The breastfeeding life is not an isolated life—and it shouldn't be. In fact, one of the best things about breastfeeding is that it is so easily integrated into other activities, even a full-time job.

If you know for a fact you will return to work, either out of necessity or simply because you love your job, you've doubtless wondered what it would be like to stay home. But even if you are deciding to be a full-time mother or start a home-based business to be near your baby, you will still need to reacquaint yourself with the outside world eventually, making contacts for your work, volunteering your time in a field that interests you, taking a class, or joining a group of other mothers and babies.

If finances permit, you could, theoretically, remain perpetually immersed in baby world, but this isn't in anyone's best interest, and it certainly is not conducive to a balanced life. Your safe, comforting, insulated world is nice, but your family isn't alone on the planet. Adult conversation and the stimulation that comes with non-baby-related work are good for your self-esteem, not to mention your health, and will help you to be a more interesting and satisfied person (and parent).

Unfortunately, getting back out there isn't as easy as just dropping the baby off at the sitter's one day and making a seamless return to the world. You have changed. A lot. Understanding how will help to ease your transition from baby world to grown-up world. And remember: you always get to go back home to your family and to the special joy of your nursing haven when the day is done.

To Work or Not to Work?

How could six weeks (or six months, or a year) go by so fast? When your maternity leave is at an end, you may feel somewhat dismayed. You aren't the same person who left that job—and now they expect you to come back?

Many women who were determined to return to work change their minds after they've had their babies. This may be possible for you, even if you hadn't really considered it before. Let's assume for now, however, that you will return to work. U.S. Labor Department statistics show that in 1996 fifty-four percent of mothers of children under one year old worked; sixty-three percent of mothers with children age two worked. Can you keep breastfeeding after going back to the office? Absolutely. In fact, the transition from full-time mother to working mother will be smoother for everyone if you don't wean yet, and coordinating breastfeeding and your job may be easier than you think.

Establishing a solid relationship with your baby before you return to work is important. Although your maternity leave may be preset at six weeks (sometimes even less), twelve weeks (three months) to six months is preferable if your employer will agree. Many companies are now willing to arrange flexible at-home work schedules for extended maternity leaves. Don't just assume your employer will say no to a flexible arrangement. If you'd like a longer period at home before returning to work, explore all the options. Remember that the 1993 Family Leave Act (see page 66) requires employers with more than fifty employees to provide up to twelve weeks of unpaid leave to employees upon the birth or adoption of a child. If you can afford it, and you want to stay home a little longer before returning to work, this is an attractive alternative.

A longer maternity leave may also mean a longer readjustment period when you do go back to work, but there are benefits to you and your baby. Optimally, breastfeeding should be well established before you return to work, and you should feel comfortable and easy about it. Also, an extended leave gives you time to nurture the crucial primary bond between mother and infant that is essential to your child's early development. But if you need or desire to return to work quickly, a high-quality relationship with your baby is certainly still possible—it will just take more planning and stamina to achieve. And, of course, continuing the breastfeeding life will only enhance that important relationship with your baby, to whom the familiar comfort and nourishment of nursing will mean all that much more now that Mom has returned to work.

Our key message to you is this: Regardless of whether you plan a brief or extended maternity leave, breastfeeding presents a distinct advantage for your baby.

The Contact Ritual That Works

The first day away from your baby will be the hardest. You might feel terrible about leaving him, or guilty for looking forward to getting out of the house. Or both. This is perfectly nat-ural. Remember that your baby, too, might be a little confused. The best way to make you both feel better is to establish a new ritual: the last thing you do before you are out the door, and the first thing you do when you return home, will be to nurse your baby.

Organize your preparation time in the morning so that you are ready to leave about thirty minutes before you actually need to be out of the house. (You'll want to wait to put on any cloth-ing that might get stained until after the nursing session.) Then take your baby to your nursing haven, relax, and focus on him completely. While he nurses, explain where you are going, and tell him you will be back. Try not to think ahead about work or do anything else during this time. This is your bonding time and you should keep it sacred. When he is done, tell him good-bye, finish dressing, and leave without a fuss. If your baby senses you are anxious or sad, he will think something is wrong. If you can't help a completely understandable crying session—very likely dur-ing the first few workdays—try to indulge after you are gone from the baby's sight. Your baby, too, may wail pitifully as you leave (especially if you make a big deal about it), but once you've been gone for ten or fifteen minutes and he realizes you can't hear him, chances are he'll be just fine. So will you.

If you can possibly organize it, either go home for lunch (or to the sitter's or daycare center) or have someone bring the baby to you for the midday feeding. If this is impossible, spend a por-tion of your lunch hour pumping your milk. This will supply your baby with milk for the next day's lunch and keep your milk supply well established. Of course, you can instruct the sitter to give your baby formula when you have to miss the midday feed-ing, but if you don't nurse or pump during the entire workday, expect some engorgement for a few days, then a decrease in your milk supply.

The best choice for pumping breastmilk at the office is the battery-operated pump, which is more effective than a manual pump. Electric pumps are the most efficient, but they are expensive and unwieldy and may be awkward to use in an office setting. Of course, you'll need to find a private place at the office where you feel comfortable pumping. If you have your own office, this may be the logical choice. Lock your door, if you can, or post a "do not disturb" sign to ensure that unwitting coworkers will not intrude uninvited. While you'll most likely want to avoid announcing to the entire office that you are pumping breastmilk every day at lunch hour, you may want to alert your supervisor, if you feel comfortable doing so. If you don't have an office, you'll need to be more creative in finding a suitable private environment; here, your supervisor may be of help and encouragement.

If you feel awkward or self-conscious about pumping at the office, that's perfectly understandable. Pumping may feel awkward to you anyway. If you know from the start of your maternity leave that you expect to return to the office and you want to continue breastfeeding after you do, practice using a pump at home so that by the time you start working again you are comfortable with it. Remember that pumping at the office will be harder psychologically than pumping at home—you won't be close to your baby, so the milk ejection reflex may be harder to stimulate. If you become experienced at home pumping, the transition to lunch hour pumping may be all that much easier to make.

It may be a good idea to buy two or three of the same blouse and keep the extras at the office in case your clothes ever become stained while pumping. Coworkers need never know. Also remember to stay hydrated during the day—don't get so carried away with a work assignment that you forget to follow the important nutritional guidelines for nursing mothers (see chapter 5).

Other employees who know you are pumping at the office may be uncomfortable with it or they may just be outright curious and ask you questions. If you are discreet and are not infringing on the space or rights of other employees, then those who are uncomfortable will have to deal with their own feelings. As for those who ask questions, be as open as you prefer to be. Breastfeeding is unknown territory for a lot of people. And you're the expert! Share in whatever way makes *you* feel comfortable. After all, these are coworkers; they're not entitled to know any more personal details about your life than you are willing to give them.

Once you've finished pumping, you will need a cold place to keep the milk. If your office has a refrigerator, great. You can store the milk in a thermos, or put plastic milk bottles in a bag, insulated bottle carrier, or a box if you are self-conscious about your milk sitting on the refrigerator shelf for all to see. If you don't have access to a refrigerator, keep a small cooler filled with ice underneath your desk or somewhere else convenient and out of the way. As soon as you get home, store the milk in the refrigerator. Then, take your baby immediately to your nursing haven and spend as long as he needs—and as long as you need—to nurse, relax, and revel in each other's presence again. For more information about how to pump and store breastmilk, see chapter 4.

The nursing ritual will keep you and your baby in touch, even as you enjoy a fulfilling life away from home. Plus, the baby will continue to receive all the benefits of your breastmilk, which can be especially helpful if he is exposed to other children in daycare. (Although he won't have immunities to any germs to which you haven't been exposed, he will probably be healthier and more resistant in general.)

Whatever you do, if you have made the decision to return to work (or if the decision has been made for you, out of necessity), *don't feel guilty!* You can be an excellent mother to your baby while working, even full-time. Make the most of your time with your baby, and don't put your job ahead of him, but enjoy your job, too. Your job is a part of you and you are good at it. Your baby will benefit from a mother who helps to support her family and who derives satisfaction from her work.

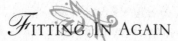FITTING IN AGAIN

Something distressing often happens to a new mother. After the first few attempts at rejoining the human race, it becomes quite clear that suddenly she seems to have absolutely nothing in common with some of her closest friends. This is, of course, natural. Motherhood changes you in unexpected ways, and friendship is often based on having interests in common with someone. You will probably find that although you are still very fond of your friends who don't have children, you won't be as interested in spending as much time with them. For one thing, spare time is a distant memory. For another, you now love talking about babies, motherhood, breastfeeding, and anything related. Of course your friends who don't have babies won't mind hearing about these things *occasionally,* but you certainly can't expect them to share your passion for size one shoes and the latest innovations in baby furniture, let alone how you are adjusting to your new breast pump!

Changing relationships are an important part of parenthood. Recognizing that you have less in common with many of your old friends and striving to cultivate relationships with other parents will help you adjust. Of course, you can certainly keep your old friends. You are a person apart from your baby, and relationships in which you can be that individual are important. So, however, are relationships where you can freely and selfishly indulge in the joys of mother-talk.

Coworkers are a different story. As we've already alluded, the work dynamics will shift when you return to the job (whether for better or worse). Some may assume you'll never be as interested in the job again now that you are a parent. Some may ask you questions about motherhood nonstop, and some may never ask you any questions and prefer that you never bring it up either. You'll need to feel your way around in the beginning to get a sense of where people in your office environment stand, and how best to interact with them. As for anyone who doubts your dedication, talent, or productivity on the job now that you're also a mother, let your professionalism speak for itself. Women all over America are successfully juggling careers and parenthood. It's a fact of life. If you find there are issues related to the workplace and motherhood that you need to talk about, seek out a trusted colleague in your office or industry who is also a working mother and ask her advice. Also rely on your breastfeeding support group. Other working mothers who are breastfeeding, and with whom you can share your feelings and experiences, if only over the telephone, will be an invaluable resource. Having a sympathetic outlet for your concerns will help you deal with them more effectively and lessen any chance for emotional confrontations on the job. Also, other women who've been through it might have creative solutions to your particular workplace issue or problem—be it related to breastfeeding or another aspect of motherhood and returning to the office.

If you find you are resentful about having to go back to work and rely on pumping breastmilk but you have no other option, you will have to reconcile these feelings. Otherwise your job, your family, your health, and the quality of your breastmilk may suffer from the stress that will be generated. Thoroughly consider your options. Is there any way at all you can work either part-time or at home? Sometimes the difficulty isn't so much in returning to work while continuing to breastfeed as it is in returning to a workplace environment that is not supportive of the breastfeeding mother. If this is happening to you, you may want to look for another position with an employer that is more accepting of breastfeeding mothers and/or is willing to offer a more flexible schedule.

WORKING AT HOME

Many women assume they'll have to return to work after they give birth. Working at home may seem like an impossible option—it involves some expenses, such as a business phone/fax line or a home computer (you may already have one!), plus a lot of motivation and organization. The range of work options for new mothers have their pros and cons, but staying at home with your baby can be a very compelling "pro." Can you afford it? Compare the costs associated with returning to your job—from transportation to childcare to a working wardrobe, etc.—to the costs of working at home. Consult a professional financial planner or accountant, if you need to. You may be able to achieve the same financial result by working fewer hours at home and taking in a lower salary doing it!

Finances aside, what kind of work could you *do* from home? If your employer were willing to extend your maternity leave with a work-at-home program, you might want to consider asking to make the situation permanent. Many women "telecommute" successfully from home, coming in to the office only for important meetings or regularly scheduled face-to-face brainstorming or reporting sessions. Some employers will allow flextime or job-sharing. If your current situation isn't flexible enough to offer a part-time or home-based arrangement, you might want to explore creating your own home-based business.

Consider what you do best. Make a list of all your skills. What education and/or training do you have? Everyone has certain things at which they excel. Are you computer literate? A really fast typist? A great writer? A superb cook? A cake decorator? A people person? Great on the telephone? An artist? A doctor? A lawyer? Do you have a flair for advertising? Do you love children (other than your own, of course)? Be as complete as possible, then examine each quality. How could you turn this quality into a money-making opportunity?

If you do decide to operate a home business, be aware that certain taxes are required, as is good record keeping. Call the Internal Revenue Service and ask for their packet of information on starting a small business. This will give you a lot of information, plus point you toward additional resources. Or you can hire someone to take care of the business end for you.

HOME-BASED BUSINESS IDEAS

◎ Provide daycare. If you love children and feel able to handle more than just your own, take in one or two other babies or small children. People are always looking for good environments for their children, and if you can provide one, you will be in demand. Check what licensing is required in your state and what other rules apply.

◎ Cater. If you love to cook, to bake, and to organize parties, consider a home catering business. Research the field. Martha Stewart started a home catering business to be able to stay home with her baby, and just look at her now! If you are good, this can also be a very lucrative field.

◎ Become a publicist. Many companies don't have the finances to hire full-time publicists, but need to promote special projects with specific time frames and budgets. If you're a public relations kind of person, promotion and publicity is a great home-based career that puts you in contact with a great variety of people and businesses.

◎ Be crafty. If you are a good crafter, consider selling your crafts. Many shops will sell crafts for you on consignment. You can also take your work to craft shows, with baby in tow. Attend a few craft shows and strike up conversations with friendly crafters. Read up on the subject.

◎ Market a gourmet product. If you make a fabulous fruitcake, marvelous muffins, or pâté to die for, consider marketing your gourmet creation. Many stores may take your packaged wares on consignment. Talk to local businesses that seem like good markets for your specialty. You may be able to branch out into wider distribution or mail order. Who knows . . . you may turn out to be the next Mrs. Fields!

◎ Freelance as an independent contractor. Many jobs, such as real estate sales, insurance sales, computer programming, writing and editing, transcription, and telemarketing, can be done from a home office. It can be even easier to get started if the field is one in which you've worked before. Talk to former (or current) employers about working on targeted projects for them at home. If you have a computer and a modem, it is easy to stay in touch with the main office. Employers who already know you are a good worker may be more willing to take a chance on you. Or take your knowledge of the industry in which you've worked and start your own company. Broaden your marketability by expanding your skills. Consider getting a real estate license, for example, or taking a course in computer graphic design. Remember, too, networking is crucial. The more connections you have, the more success you will have.

◎ Deliver newspapers. Just for kids? Not necessarily. You can make a fairly good supplemental income if your area needs carriers, and you can take your baby with you in the car.

◎ Get into sales. Several large companies (you know who they are) employ people to work on their own time. Many advertise "no door-to-door," and you can develop a customer base solely over the phone or through people you already know. If you enjoy people and are friendly and outgoing, you might really enjoy sales. However, be aware that you are sometimes required to purchase products for resale out of your own pocket. If you are talented at sales, you could do very well marketing Christmas gifts, Tupperware, cosmetics, or herbal remedies, for example. If you aren't comfortable selling, you probably won't enjoy it enough to make a living. And don't sell a product you don't like—you won't feel good about it, and you probably won't be successful.

⊚ Consult. If you are a respected professional in any field (law, medicine, business, computers, engineering), you can make an excellent living as a consultant. Companies hire you as a sort of temporary employee to advise them on particular projects. Pay can be very high if you are good. It can be difficult to get started, but once you have cultivated a few good clients, you are in business. Much of the work can be done on your own time, and when you do need to be at an office or job site, you can hire an occasional baby-sitter.

Lots of books are available about starting your own business. Start your research now. Read everything you can on the subject. Network. Talk to everyone you can find who has experience in any area you think might interest you. Contact the National Association of Women Business Owners (800-55-NAWBO). The more you learn, the more possible self-employment will seem to you. If you are highly motivated to stay home, can work hard without constant directions from an employer, and can cultivate a lot of self-confidence, you can do it! And you'll have the freedom to integrate the breastfeeding life easily into your daily working schedule.

The National Foundation for Women Business Owners, affiliated with NAWBO, reports that in 1996 there were nearly eight million women-owned businesses in the United States, accounting for thirty-six percent of all firms in the country. The foundation also reports that, in the same year, an estimated 3.5 million home-based businesses owned by women provided full- or part-time employment to fourteen million people. Working at home isn't a far-fetched idea, it's a reality for more and more Americans. If you think working at home could be the answer for you, look into it—don't just assume a home-based solution is out of reach.

FATHER ALERT!

*B*E *U*NITED, *N*OT *D*IVIDED

After you and your partner have made a decision about whether or not she will return to work, the best thing you can do for her is to stick by her, no matter what. New mothers receive a lot of criticism about any work-related decision they make. You wouldn't believe some of the comments they hear! "I can't believe you're actually going to put that precious little baby into a *daycare center!*" "You just stay home all day? What do you *do?*" "Don't you think it would be healthier for that child to get some social interaction?" "A breastfeeding woman doesn't belong in an office." It really is relentless. It will be hard for her to escape occasional bouts of guilt no matter what path you've chosen as a family. She is bound to waver, sooner or later, unless you step in as the valiant supporter you are. Some version of "We're really happy with the decisions we've made for our family," spoken with an authoritative, polite but "mind-your-own-business" tone will do wonders, especially for your partner's confidence in herself and in you. In private, too, remind her, when she inevitably wonders if she is doing the right thing, that you will both make your situation work for your family. If you fuel her doubts, she'll only lose confidence. If you support her role, either as working mother, stay-at-home mother, or home-working mother, she can do anything!

*L*IVING THE *B*REASTFEEDING *L*IFE

Whether you decide to stay at home as a full-time mother, work full- or part-time in an office setting, or start your own home-based business, you can continue to breastfeed your baby for as long as you choose to.

Returning to work doesn't mean you'll be forced to abandon nursing. Nursing while continuing your career can be a wonderful way to reaffirm your commitment to your child as you reenter the workplace and reconnect with your professional identity. You don't have to choose one identity—mother or employee—over the other!

If you're staying at home with your baby, a looser schedule that allows you a more independent existence is not incompatible with breastfeeding. Just because you're breastfeeding doesn't mean you have to stay at home all day every day.

If, however, you do return to work and decide that the demands of working and breastfeeding are too difficult—for example, pumping at the office just doesn't work for you—continue to breastfeed for as long as you can before beginning the weaning process. Weaning your baby abruptly when you return to work may heighten his sense of disorientation and loss. A gradual weaning will make the transition easier for both of you.

We are living in an exciting time when our society's gender roles are changing and women have so many new choices. These choices can often make life confusing, but also wonderful! You really *do* have the freedom to choose the path that works best for you as an individual, and for your family as a unit. Breastfeeding executive breaking through the glass ceiling: great! Breastfeeding full-time mother: fantastic! Breastfeeding work-at-home entrepreneur: hooray! We congratulate you all. You've all chosen to give breastfeeding a try, which gives your baby the healthy advantages of breastmilk that will last her a lifetime. And your examples will encourage other women to give breastfeeding a try too.

10

MAKING THE DECISION TO WEAN

WHEN TO WEAN

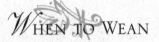

*Y*OU may decide to wean when your baby is one year old, if you become pregnant again, or when people begin to hint that it's "about time." To get the maximum health benefit for your baby, many pediatricians recommend breastfeeding for the first year, if you can. If you make the decision to wean sooner than the first year, it may mean extra effort on your part to make the transition from your breast to bottle or cup as smooth and nontraumatic for your baby as possible.

EARLY WEANING

If you do need to wean your baby before she is necessarily ready to do so on her own, the process is simple. First, make sure your nursing schedule is regular. Nurse her at the same times each day. Be as consistent as possible. If she wants to nurse before the proper time, tell her to wait, then distract her. Next, every two to three weeks or so, drop one of the feedings at the breast. Start with the feedings in the middle of the day (morning and night feedings are usually the last to go because a baby uses these to gear up and wind down).

WHO'S READY TO WEAN?

Look for the following signs in your baby and in yourself, which all signal a readiness to move beyond the breastfeeding experience. If any of these signs occur before nine to twelve months, they are probably due to other factors and do not signal a readiness to wean. In this case, talk to your doctor; also consider your baby's environment—she may be on a nursing strike (see chapter 6).

◉ Your baby nurses for extremely short periods of time and is easily distracted, constantly pulling away to look around, sit up, or squirm away.

◉ Your milk supply has dwindled significantly (this can happen when the baby doesn't nurse very often, nurses lazily, or nurses without interest, consequently failing to signal the milk ejection reflex).

◉ Your baby displays an apparent impatience or indifference to nursing, and sometimes has to be coerced to nurse.

◉ Your baby seems to want to nurse out of boredom, and then only for a short time.

◉ You are getting tired of nursing, and your baby can sense it.

◉ Your baby has significantly increased his intake of milk and food. He drinks out of a bottle or cup with no problem.

◉ Life is normal, unstressful, and regular. Everyone is happy and healthy. The environment is ripe to try something new.

When the time of the dropped feeding comes around, be sure to engage your child in some interesting, stimulating activity. Offer her formula, milk, or juice in a cup and a snack. If you start her on a bottle, that will be one more thing from which you'll have to wean her, although many parents find that bottles make weaning from the breast an easier transition. (If you are weaning your child from your breast very early in her life in favor of formula bottle-feeding, of course, you will go through a second weaning process to move your child from the bottle to a cup when she gets a little older.) The feeding time will probably pass without her even noticing, but if she does cry and make a fuss, don't worry too much. She'll learn. Drop feedings one by one until your baby has forgotten about them or, at least, is able to do without them.

If your baby is extremely resistant to weaning, she may truly not be ready. You can persist, but remember that babies do have sucking needs. If she doesn't suck her thumb or a bottle, she may be feeling a profound loss. If her resistance is particularly strong or particularly hard on you, consider whether you really need to wean her yet. If weaning isn't a necessity, why not let her be done with it at her own pace? Many women who decide to wean their children change their minds once they've attempted the process, and return to breastfeeding, committed to a child-led approach. If you are sure you do want to wean her, however, be especially affectionate and comforting to her during this transition. Also, engage Dad's help. He can be affectionate without subjecting the baby to the temptation of the unattainable breast so close at hand.

CHILD-LED WEANING

A more satisfying way to wean, if your circumstances and inclinations allow, is to let your child make her own decision to give up the breast. Although some people might tell you that child-led weaning isn't good because it gives your child too much control, or because she won't *ever* wean on her own, be assured that neither is true. Child-led weaning bestows a wonderful gift upon your little one: she will never be denied the security and special comfort she receives at your breast; instead, she will grow past this need at her own pace. And child-led weaning does involve plenty of intervention, guidance, and reassuring cues from Mom. It is anything but a passive process on the part of the parents.

Babies growing into toddlerhood are demanding, inquisitive, and exhausting little creatures. It is all too easy to put them to the breast in lieu of another game of "swing me in a circle" or "throw this and watch Mommy pick it up again." Also, when the well of ideas runs dry and you don't know what else to do with your toddler, you may routinely put him to the breast out of boredom. He may want to nurse for the same reasons; if he can't find anything more stimulating to do, he might as well nurse again. You'll want to keep from falling into this trap as you and your growing child begin the child-led weaning process in earnest.

The best way to approach life with a toddler is to concentrate on his amazing learning process. Keeping him busy, stimulated, and interested is often the key to his decision to wean himself. Instead of concentrating on weaning and withholding the breast, concentrate on engaging your child's interest in his environment. The more the world fascinates him, the less often he'll have the time or the inclination to sit in one place for very long, even if that place is cuddled on your lap. During times of stress, illness, or insecurity, though, he may temporarily regress and want to nurse more often. By allowing him to nurse under these circumstances, he will feel secure in the knowledge that the comfort of nursing is still available to him. Often, this will paradoxically contribute to the gradual elimination of his desire to nurse at all. He will feel increasingly confident as he realizes that his mother will always be there in times of trouble and that stressful events aren't made more stressful because nursing is denied.

The age at which your child will choose to wean varies immensely. At about nine months, many babies suddenly lose interest in nursing. External distractions have become so much more compelling that breastfeeding is old hat, and the baby becomes ready to move on to bigger and better things. On the other hand, don't *assume* a nine-month-old who is reluctant to nurse is ready to wean. First, rule out other factors that might be causing a nursing strike (see chapter 6). If your family is in a period of change or is experiencing a particularly stressful time, your baby may become reluctant to nurse. Spend a few weeks conducting nursing sessions in a quiet room without any distractions. Concentrate on nursing (in other words, don't do ten other things at the same time, no matter how busy you are). If your baby's lack of interest persists, she may indeed be ready for the cup.

If your baby nurses energetically right through the ninth month and you have decided to let him wean himself, you may end up nursing through toddlerhood. Of course, a three-year-old nurses far less often than a six-month-old or even a one- or two-year-old, frequently only once every few days. A child who can communicate with language, although not able to reason with adult logic, will be able to understand if you tell her that nursing is allowed only in certain situations, but not in others, such as in public. Limiting times during which nursing is allowed without denying nursing altogether can be an effective way to encourage the weaning process. Invariably, if a child is denied something categorically, she will want it even more. If she knows she may nurse (within the parameters you have established, such as when you are at home), she will only nurse when she really needs it.

The weaning process becomes an important life-lesson for your child in respecting boundaries—and also in trust. Your behavior must be consistent, warm and supportive, and straightforward so that the message you convey to your child will be understood clearly. As psychoanalyst Carl Jung wrote in *The Integration of the Personality*, "If there is anything that we wish to change in the child, we should first examine it and see whether it is not something that could be better changed in ourselves." If your child seems confused or weaning is a difficult emotional experience for both of you, take a look at whether you may be sending some mixed signals and adjust your behavior accordingly.

If you decide to let your child wean at his own pace, stick with this decision. If you find yourself apologizing or feeling defensive about your decision, remember that nursing is the most natural thing in the world, and you don't owe anyone an explanation. If your baby has had enough of the breast at nine months, move on to new activities. If she seems to need and love the security of the breast until she is three or four, grant her this security and cherish the cuddle time, which will, all too soon, be just a memory.

Breastfeeding Past the First Year

For many mothers, that "one year mark" is the understood time to wean. After that year is over, shouldn't you, well . . . stop? Isn't breastfeeding a child who can talk a little strange? If she can ask for it, should she be able to have it?

Why not? Breastfeeding a toddler serves many of the same functions as breastfeeding an infant. Although the nutritional content of breastmilk declines after the first year, toddlers can benefit from the continued supply of vitamins and immunities they receive from mother's milk. But this change in your milk is natural; in toddlerhood, breastmilk is, of course, no longer the primary part of a baby's diet. At this stage, nursing is more like an emotionally supportive, personalized, immune-boosting vitamin supplement! (Don't you wish we could all have such a supplement?) And toddlers don't really need to suck in the profound way they did through the first year. At a time when your baby is testing his wings, venturing out into the world, and moving, so it seems, further and further away from you, you will cherish those precious moments when he runs back into your arms, cuddles, and nurses. The world is a stimulating, exciting, and sometimes

THE PROS AND CONS OF NURSING PAST THE FIRST YEAR

PROS

◎ It's a great way to stay in touch with an active toddler.

◎ It's also an unbeatable source of nutrition and immunities for your toddler.

◎ Your toddler's emotional needs will be met through the comfort of nursing when he needs to.

◎ Letting your baby wean when *she* is ready, rather than when *you* are ready, eases her more naturally into the next phase of development. You'll both feel better about it.

◎ Nursing is an excellent way to calm a baby when he is tired, fussy, or sick.

◎ A sick toddler may not be able to keep down any food but mother's milk.

◎ All toddlers are clingy. Breastfeeding doesn't make them more so—it makes them less so because they feel confident and secure.

◎ You really enjoy nursing and you don't feel ready to end this special communion with your baby.

◎ You may be able to put off menstruation for several years! (Suppressing ovulation may help protect against ovarian cancer, too.)

◎ Sometimes it's fun to be a rebel!

CONS

◉ Sometimes it *isn't* fun to be a rebel. People may criticize you or give you strange looks if you nurse in public or mention that you are still nursing your child.

◉ You may feel like your body belongs to a two-and-a-half-foot-tall dictator.

◉ It can be easier to wean a nine-to-twelve-month-old who is developing an active interest in the world than a stubborn, headstrong toddler who is (relatively) set in his ways.

◉ If you weaned her, you'd be able to eat and drink whatever you want. (But remember, her eyes will be on you as you reach for that box of donuts, setting a dubious high-fat example. Try to keep your healthy eating habits firmly in place!)

◉ You may fall into the trap of doing nothing with your child but nursing at a time when she can benefit from many other types of interaction with you.

◉ If you become pregnant again, nursing may become irritating due to increasingly sensitive breasts (although not always, and it can be done).

◉ You love your child, but to be quite honest, you are just plain *sick* of breastfeeding! You are ready to move on, and you suspect your baby is, too.

overwhelming place for a toddler. Nursing allows him temporarily to stop the bombardment on his senses and regroup. Then, off he'll go again. There is no good evidence that breastfeeding past the first year is emotionally harmful to your child.

Although women in many other countries breastfeed toddlers, here in the United States, the practice is considered unusual, and finding support can be difficult. As Americans become increasingly educated about the benefits of breastfeeding, nursing toddlers may become more common, but unfortunately, the practice is still somewhat of a rarity, particularly after age two.

If you are still straddling the fence on whether or not to breastfeed past the first year, please realize that the most important issue to consider is whether or not your child seems ready to wean. Some one-year-olds have no problem relinquishing the breast, and many do it with barely a nudge, especially when other activities are regularly offered as an interesting alternative. Other toddlers seem extremely attached to nursing well beyond the first year (and there's nothing wrong with that). Every baby has her own personality, and you know your baby better than anyone. Not even your doctor can possibly know as well as you whether your baby is ready to wean or not. If you and your baby still enjoy nursing, there is absolutely no reason to give it up. Letting your baby decide when she is ready to wean can be an immensely satisfying choice for a breastfeeding family to make.

PREGNANT AND STILL BREASTFEEDING?

Many women decide to wean their babies when they become pregnant again, and many doctors recommend this, too. If breastfeeding while pregnant makes you uncomfortable, either physically or emotionally, and if your toddler seems ready, by all means, start the weaning process. Don't feel you have to wean if you aren't ready, however.

A pregnant and breastfeeding mother has to be careful to eat enough nutritious food, especially adequate protein and calcium. A high fluid intake is also helpful. In fact, all the things a pregnant woman should be doing for her health pretty much coincide with what a nursing mother should do. Just be sure to eat. Although studies are inconclusive, if your nutrient intake is insuf-

Six Answers to the Inevitable Question: "Are You Still Nursing Your Child?"

- ◎ "I'm certainly curious about when she'll be ready to wean, but we're in no hurry."

- ◎ "Far be it for me to deprive him of the perfect food!"

- ◎ "Yes, it's such a comfort to have that time together since she has become so independent."

- ◎ "I've decided to let *him* decide when he is ready to stop."

- ◎ "Of course! Nursing is much better for his teeth than a bottle, but we're practicing with the cup, too."

- ◎ And to those for whom you feel no detailed explanation is warranted (you certainly don't owe an explanation to *anyone*), a calm and self-assured, "Yes."

ficient, your body may deprive the fetus of nutrients in favor of continued lactation. As long as you are eating well, however, this won't happen and you needn't worry.

You can even continue to breastfeed your toddler once your new baby is born. This is called tandem nursing, and it is relatively uncommon simply because to many women, it just seems so complicated! It can certainly be a good experience, however, especially for the toddler who feels left out when the new sibling arrives. Tandem nursing can actually help to establish a good milk supply for the new infant, and your toddler may enjoy the renewed and prodigious flow of milk. Don't be worried that your toddler will get all the milk. You'll always make more. It's best to feed your infant first, however, and then let your toddler have a turn (or, if you are really coordinated, you can offer each child a breast). Just as a lot of people have limited experience with breastfeeding, even fewer people have experience with tandem nursing and they may have a hard time with the concept. If the idea of tandem nursing makes *you* uncomfortable, you are certainly not "required" to try it. Your toddler will be just fine if you wean him before your baby is born. On the other hand, if tandem nursing works for your family, don't let anyone discourage you.

If you do wean your toddler before you next baby is born, be sure to give him a lot of attention and love. Some toddlers who are weaned will ask or attempt to nurse again when your new baby is nursing. Jealousy is natural, of course. Let him try it if you are comfortable. He probably just wants a quick taste and will then move on. Otherwise, tell him he is too big for that now, then quickly reassure him in other ways. Give him lots of hugs and kisses, and allot special time each day with just the two of you. He must know that the end of nursing is in no way an end to physical closeness between the two of you.

Whenever possible, let your toddler help you care for the new baby. He can bring you diapers, hand you the baby powder, or help you rub in the baby lotion. He can lend a hand drying off the baby after a bath, and you can make it his job to sing, dance, and otherwise entertain the new baby. You will be laying the groundwork for a healthy sibling relationship. In addition, a confident toddler who feels loved and appreciated will be less likely to be resentful of his new sibling's breastfeeding relationship with Mom. Making an effort to bring siblings together in this way is a key to holistic living—your family will be learning to work together and each child will learn mutual respect and affection. Healthy family relationships encourage health in general.

THE WEANING BLUES QUIZ

You have to wean, or you want to wean, or your baby seems to want to wean, and you've started the weaning process—but maybe things aren't going the way you envisioned. Every mom and every baby is different, so every weaning experience is unique. There are some typical problems and tendencies, however. Take this quiz to determine your weaning profile, then read on for tips about how to make weaning easier for you and your baby (or why you might consider postponing a bit longer). Pick the one best answer for each question.

1. The main reason I want or need to wean is:

   A. *I have to go back to work, I have to be away from the baby for a while, I'm pregnant again, or I have some medical problem that makes nursing difficult or impossible.*
   B. *My baby doesn't seem very interested anymore. He keeps stopping to look around or wants to do other things, and he eats plenty of solid foods.*
   C. *My friends and relatives keep hinting that I've been nursing more than long enough, and I wonder if my child is getting too old, even though I still enjoy nursing.*

2. When my child wants to nurse and I don't let her, the worst thing that happens is:

   A. *I feel incredibly guilty and sad.*
   B. *She gets very upset, frustrated, even angry.*
   C. *She is mildly persistent but easily distracted to something else.*

3. Weaning has affected me primarily:

   A. *Physically. I've had intense mood swings, been extra irritable, experienced hair loss, had sore breasts, or even experienced a fever and flu-like symptoms.*
   B. *Emotionally. I feel incredibly sad, like I've experienced a loss.*
   C. *In a positive way. I've experienced some physical symptoms, but I'm so glad to have my body back, and to see my baby's blooming independence.*

4. The worst part about weaning has been:

   A. *Feelings of uselessness. Does my baby need me anymore?*
   B. *Guilt at stopping before my baby chose to stop.*
   C. *Saying good-bye to a meaningful stage of parenting.*

5. My child has responded to my weaning efforts by:

   A. *Becoming extremely persistent about wanting to nurse constantly. He grabs at my clothes, continually asks to nurse (if a toddler), or squirms and cries more than usual.*
   B. *Acting surprisingly mature, finding new things to do and new ways to cuddle, although when he's had a bad day or falls down, his first reaction is to want to nurse.*
   C. *Acting uncomfortable or sad around me, as if he thinks I've betrayed him.*

6. My method of weaning is:

   A. *Sudden—we went cold turkey.*
   B. *To quit for a while, then start again, then quit again, then start again.*
   C. *Gradual—we cut down one feeding at a time.*

7. When my child does nurse, it seems to be:

   A. *Out of boredom.*
   B. *An intense time for her.*
   C. *Out of habit.*

8. The first time my child didn't ask to nurse at a regular feeding, such as going to sleep on his own without nursing or going straight to the table for breakfast when he wakes up, I felt:

   A. *Proud.*
   B. *Rejected.*
   C. *Unsettled, as if my child has given up trying to get what he wants.*

9. My own feelings about weaning that bother me the most are:

   A. *I feel like I'm not a good mother because I decided to wean rather than letting my child decide. Will she hold it against me? Does she feel like I rejected her?*
   B. *I feel selfish about wanting my body back, or about not wanting to nurse when I go back to work.*
   C. *I feel uncomfortable that I gave in to pressure from books or friends or relatives and weaned before my child was ready.*

10. My plans for developing my relationship with my child, after weaning, are:

    A. *To try to get over my feelings of loss and guilt.*
    B. *To show my child how to bond with me, physically, without nursing—through hugs, kisses, and lots of cuddling.*
    C. *To concentrate on replacing nursing with something else—a bottle, a pacifier, a thumb, anything to make it easier.*

Using the following key, count how many I's, II's, and III's you have:

1. A-I, B-II, C-III
2. A-III, B-I, C-II
3. A-I, B-III, C-II
4. A-III, B-I, C-II
5. A-I, B-II, C-III
6. A-I, B-III, C-II
7. A-II, B-I, C-III
8. A-II, B-III, C-I
9. A-III, B-II, C-I
10. A-III, B-II, C-I

I: _____ II: _____ III: _____

If you chose mostly I's: Maybe you had to wean, or maybe you thought you wanted to wean, or maybe friends and relatives were pressuring you to wean, but now that you've done it, you're second-guessing yourself. Your baby doesn't seem ready and you feel bad about it, or at least a little guilty. Listen to your feelings. If you feel like weaning was "wrong," it was probably done prematurely. If it's possible, you might consider resuming breastfeeding. Even if you've stopped for a few days or a few weeks, you can start again, if you are still producing milk (if you've stopped lactating, you may even be able to start again with some persistance). If your baby wasn't ready to wean, he'll probably be glad to pick right back up where he left off. Remember that, even if you've had to return to work, nursing can still be a wonderful way to bond with your baby before you leave in the morning and after you get home. If, however, you've had to wean out of some necessity, try to wean gradually, if possible. Gradual weaning is easier on your baby and on your body (sudden weaning will cause sudden hormone fluctuations in you). Then, move on. Your baby will be fine. Even if he wasn't ready, he'll adjust, as long as he's receiving sufficient nutrition, and lots of extra cuddling from you. Nursing isn't the only way babies and moms bond, so put your weaning experience behind you and concentrate on loving your child. Your child may actually be having less of a hard time than you are with the weaning process. Are you projecting your feelings onto your child?

If you chose mostly II's: Things are going well. You waited until your baby was showing signs she was ready, and then you initiated weaning gradually. Sometimes you'll feel sad about it. You may experience physical symptoms of weaning, such as sore breasts or mood swings, because even when you are ready to wean, your hormone levels will fluctuate due to weaning. You may feel guilty when your child wants to nurse and you persuade her to do something else instead. You also may feel guilty about being happy to be done with breastfeeding. All that is normal.

What's important is that you and your baby have made the step together, and in general things are going well. Don't give in to the urge to lapse back into nursing once you've been successful. You and your baby have moved to a new level in your relationship, and you can always look back fondly on the nursing stage.

If you chose mostly III's: Chances are, weaning has been much harder on you than it has been on your child. He may have been nursing purely out of habit, or because you seemed to enjoy it and it was an easy way to bond with you. Maybe you feel like you won't be as necessary in his life if you wean him. Nothing could be further from the truth. Weaning signals a new stage in your baby's life, when you become even more important as a role model, teacher, world tour guide, and source of unconditional love. If your child is having trouble with weaning, it may be because you are sending mixed signals. You want to wean, but then you feel so terrible about the loss of that closeness that you try to nurse again. Then you try to take it away again. If your baby is ready to wean and you're not, start out trying to nurse only when your baby wants to, not when you want to, to get you back in touch with what your baby really needs. Remember, you're the adult and the one (along with your partner) who's responsible for making decisions in your child's best interest. Recognize your new role and embrace it. If he is ready, your baby will follow your lead, and he won't hold weaning against you.

Moving Past the Breastfeeding Life

You've done it. You've weaned your baby. Whether he is nine months, one year, or three years old, you have entered the next stage of parenthood. Breastfeeding will soon be a memory, but a vivid and cherished one. You may experience temporary engorgement if you wean too quickly. Dropping feedings very gradually will be helpful. Even if you find your baby has self-weaned fairly quickly and you are experiencing pain, know that it will soon pass. Occasional pumping or manually expressing a little milk to relieve engorgement can help, but don't pump too often, as this will maintain your milk supply.

Sometimes, weaning moms may feel slightly feverish or get a clogged milk duct or a breast infection due to the engorgement. Also, weaning will cause an adjustment in your hormones, which may cause mood swings or a feeling of melancholy. If your period hasn't already started or is sporadic, it will probably recommence or become more regular again within a few months. If you think you have a breast infection or engorgement is very uncomfortable, talk to your doctor about possible therapies.

During the time of weaning you also may experience mild depression, which may be caused or exacerbated by your hormonal shift. You are leaving behind an important part of parenthood and, although you know it is time, the thought of never nursing your baby again may be upsetting. This is completely normal.

Just remember that weaning is actually a step toward the development of a new complexity in your relationship with your baby. She is growing up, but she still needs you, both physically and emotionally. She needs you for hugs and kisses and cuddling. She needs you for words of encouragement, instruction, guidance, and affection. You are her mother, and that means quite a lot beyond "bearer of the breasts." You have given your baby life. You have nourished your baby in the best way possible. Now your baby is a child, ready for you to guide her with love into the future.

Dad can join you more fully and more meaningfully now, too. Your parenting can be truly a complementary effort. And don't worry about losing your baby too soon. Together, you will guide your child into the future and he can go forward with confidence, secure in the knowledge that you are standing behind him, just in case he needs you.

FATHER ALERT!

WHY WELCOME WEANING?

At long last, your child is weaning. This signals a new stage in your relationship. You are soon to become a much more significant force in your baby's life. Yes, that's a good thing! Yes, that's also a scary thing. When the baby no longer depends on breastfeeding, he will be able to concentrate on developing relationships based on more complex interactions. You will become a role model. He will go through stages where he is very attached to you and imitates everything you do. Make sure you are worthy of imitation!

And don't forget your partner. Weaning can be emotionally difficult for mothers, even when they *want* to wean and are tired of breastfeeding. You've observed the intense bonding and closeness between your partner and your baby since birth. That's about to change. She may experience sadness, even grief. The best thing you can do is listen. Let her talk about it. Don't worry about solving the "problem" of her sadness. It will solve itself. Don't worry if her feelings seem contradictory. Instead, be supportive and tell her how glad you are that she gave your baby such an important foundation for his health and emotional well-being. Plan your baby's toddlerhood together. Discuss parenting issues that will soon arise, such as discipline, house rules, school. Help her focus on the future. You have many parental adventures ahead of you, which you will experience together. The more involved you are in your child's life, and the more united your parental front, the happier and more secure your child will be.

And remember, the best thing you can do for your child is to love each other. Now more than ever, you must nourish and cultivate your relationship.

Your family is growing and changing. Continue to steer each other toward health and happiness with respect, affection, and love. Breastfeeding was an auspicious beginning for the child— and the family—you have created. If you live the rest of your lives according to the same natural, simple, holistic practices you have followed while living the breastfeeding life, your family can't help but thrive.

MINI FAMILY COOKBOOK

*T*HIS mini family cookbook will make your life easier. Each section—based on different baby stages—presents recipes for family meals or snacks that include baby food preparation, so the baby can eat what the family eats, or a modified version.

Eating in harmony with the seasons will provide you with food that is more nutritious because it hasn't been stored for months or shipped from far away. Buying food at farmers' markets, produce stands, or grocery stores that stock local produce and/or organically grown food will provide your family with the highest quality ingredients. Some recipes guide you regarding the season for which they are appropriate. All meals containing meat are adaptable for vegetarian families. And remember, the quality of your meals, not to mention the quality of your breastmilk, depends on the quality of your food. Whenever possible, choose whole foods, natural foods, organic foods, and foods grown close to your home (or better yet, in your own backyard!).

GREAT MEALS TO COOK AND FREEZE

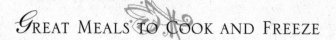

While you're waiting for your baby to arrive, plan ahead by cooking some nutritious meals that freeze easily. That way, you'll be sure to have quick, easy, and healthy meals you can count on. You'll have less stress, more time to focus on establishing your breastfeeding relationship with your baby, and the nutrient-rich food that will ensure high-quality breastmilk.

Of course, these meals are a good idea anytime. You may find you come to rely on them as the hectic schedules of parenthood put your time at a premium. You want to have the best diet possible!

HEARTY SPAGHETTI CASSEROLE

*I*F YOU choose not to use meat in this delicious casserole, add an additional one or two cups chopped vegetables, such as cubed zucchini, butternut or yellow squash, extra mushrooms, broccoli florets, red bell peppers, or whatever you like. You can also substitute ziti or any other pasta for the spaghetti.

    1 lb. spaghetti
    1 lb. ground turkey breast or lean ground beef (optional)
    1/2 cup sliced turkey kielbasa (optional)
    2 tablespoons vegetable oil (if not using meat)
    1 medium onion, chopped

2 *cloves garlic, diced or put through a garlic press*
1 *cup mushrooms, sliced*
1/2 *green bell pepper, diced*
1 *carrot, grated*
1 *8-oz. can tomato sauce plus one can of water*
1 *6-oz. can tomato paste plus one can of water*
1 *teaspoon each dried basil and oregano, crushed (or use 2*
    teaspoons each of the fresh herbs)
1 *4-oz. can sliced black olives (optional, but yummy!)*
2 *cups shredded mozzarella cheese*

Break spaghetti into bite-sized pieces, then cook the spaghetti in a large pot of boiling, salted water, according to package directions. Rinse well and drain in a colander, then set aside.

Brown the ground turkey or beef and drain. Return to heat. (Or, if not using meat, heat two tablespoons vegetable oil.) Add the onion, garlic, and, optionally, the kielbasa. Cook and stir until the onion is translucent but not brown and the kielbasa is lightly browned. Add the mushrooms, bell pepper, and carrot. Cook until green pepper is soft. Add the tomato sauce plus a can full of water, then the tomato paste plus a can full of water. Add the basil and oregano, and stir in the olives. Bring the mixture to a boil, then cook covered on low heat for one hour. Uncover and cook for an additional hour, or until the sauce is thick.

(Note: you don't need to add salt. The kielbasa and olives (and cheese) add enough. If you leave these out, you can add up to one teaspoon of salt to boost the flavor, or just go salt-free.)

Remove the sauce from the heat. Add spaghetti and mix well. Spray a 9" × 13" baking pan or casserole with nonstick cooking spray. Layer half the spaghetti mixture, half the cheese, half the spaghetti mixture, and the remaining cheese. Allow to cool at room temperature for about 30 minutes (not over an hour). Cover with lid or foil and freeze.

To cook, remove from freezer and bake, covered with foil, at 400 degrees for 45 minutes. Remove foil and cook for an additional 15 minutes or until bubbly and hot in the center. Serve with homemade garlic bread made with olive oil and fresh, pressed garlic, and a salad. Serves eight (or good for two meals for a family of four).

FREEZABLE FRENCH TOAST BRUNCH

FRENCH TOAST

1 loaf good French bread
8 eggs
1 cup milk (whatever "strength" you like)
¼ cup unsalted butter or cooking oil (you can use cooking spray to save calories, though the taste isn't quite as delicious)

The night before, slice the loaf of French bread into ½-inch to 1-inch slices. Spread them out on a cutting board or other clean surface (out of reach of pets!). Cover with a towel.

The next morning, break all the eggs into a large mixing bowl. Mix well. Add milk and mix until the mixture looks uniform.

Heat a skillet, then melt one tablespoon of the butter or

cooking oil. While the oil is heating, float a few pieces of bread in the egg mixture, flipping to coat both sides well. Let the bread sit in the egg mixture for at least thirty seconds, as long as two minutes. When the skillet is hot, fry the soaked bread on both sides. Make sure the skillet isn't too hot, or the outside will be overdone and the inside raw. When golden brown, transfer with a spatula to a paper towel. When cool, move the toast to a cookie sheet. Repeat with the remaining slices of bread.

When all the bread is cooked and spread out on cookie sheets, put the sheets in the freezer. Freeze for at least four hours, then remove bread slices to a large freezer bag. Yield: about eight servings (depends on the size of your bread loaf and the hunger of your family!).

Tasty, occasional option: You don't want to be in the habit of sugar-coating this nutritious breakfast, but an occasional splurge for a birthday or other festive occasion won't hurt, and this French toast "dress-up" is delicious. After you have fried each piece of toast, dip both sides in a mixture of ½ cup sugar and 1 tablespoon cinnamon, spread on a plate. Freeze as directed.

FRUIT SAUCE

4 cups fresh, ripe fruit (whatever is in season or looks good,
such as peaches, nectarines, apricots, apples, strawberries,
raspberries, blueberries, cranberries, etc.—organic will taste
better) or frozen, defrosted fruit (with no sugar added)
1 can frozen apple juice concentrate
¼ cup cornstarch mixed with 2 tablespoons water
cinnamon (optional, if it seems to go with your choice of fruit)

Peel fruit and cut into chunks (not berries; they're fine the way they are, except core the strawberries). Combine fruit and apple juice concentrate in a medium saucepan. Cook over medium heat for about 30 minutes or until fruit is soft. Allow to cool slightly, then puree the mixture in a blender. Return to saucepan and stir in cornstarch mixture. Heat again over medium-high heat, stirring frequently, until sauce boils. Stir in the optional cinnamon. Allow to bubble, stirring constantly, until sauce is thick. Remove from heat. Allow to cool. Transfer to freezable container or freezer bag. Label and freeze. Yield: about eight generous servings.

Option: Buy a package of brown-and-serve turkey sausage or vegetarian breakfast sausage, and store with French toast for an easy-cook or microwave addition.

To serve, remove all freezer bags. Arrange French toast in a single layer on cookie sheets or baking pans (just take out as much as you need). Bake in a preheated 400-degree oven for 30 minutes or until you can hear it all sizzling just a little. While it is cooking, cook optional sausage in the microwave oven or on the stove. Remove fruit sauce and heat in the microwave for 3 minutes (or until defrosted and warm), stirring once a minute, or defrost the fruit sauce the day before and warm it in a saucepan.

Helpful hint for later, or for big brother or sister: French toast cut into small cubes and coated with fruit sauce makes a great toddler finger food.

SEASONAL SMOOTHIES FOR THE BREASTFEEDING MOTHER — AND BABY, TOO!

Smoothies are a wonderful invention. Thick and creamy like milkshakes but with no sugar and little if any fat, they are a

FATHER ALERT!

GET COOKIN'!

Who says you can't do some of the cooking? If you're an accomplished cook, you probably won't need these helpful tips on finding your way around the kitchen. But if you do, here they are. We promise that if you cook for her, she'll love it. You will, too.

◎ Clean as you go along.

◎ Start with simple recipes. The more you learn, the better you will get, but if you start with something too complicated and it doesn't work, you may turn against cooking forever. If you don't know the difference between mixing, stirring, blending, whipping, and pureeing, don't worry. Cookbooks have this information, and so may your partner (if she is the cook in the family). Or call up a kitchen-savvy friend. The point is, if you don't know, ask.

◎ Take out all the ingredients and all the proper bowls, measuring devices, and cooking pans before you start even the first step of the recipe. Then you will be sure you have everything you need and you won't get stuck without eggs or a tablespoon at a crucial point in preparation.

◎ Don't assume that if an ingredient is almost like another ingredient, they can be substituted for one another. Baking power and baking soda are not interchangeable. Neither are evaporated milk, sweetened condensed milk, and regular milk, or all-purpose flour, cake flour, and bread flour. Most cookbooks have substitution lists that tell you what you can substitute when you don't have something. If you wing it, the recipe may not work.

◉ If weather permits, experiment with outdoor grilling, a fun way to prepare a meal that can be as simple or elaborate as you make it.

◉ As often as you can, use whole, natural, organic, fresh ingredients. They are healthier and taste better.

◉ And remember: some of the world's greatest chefs are men!

healthy and satisfying snack, dessert, or even quick breakfast. Always use plain, unsweetened yogurt, fat-free, lowfat, or regular. Milk can be whole, low-fat, or skim, depending on whether the smoothie is for you or your baby. Keep a supply of frozen bananas on hand so you can make a smoothie whenever you crave one. Always buy more bananas than you will eat. When the last few get very ripe and the skins are mostly black, peel them, wrap them individually in plastic or freezer bags, and store in the freezer for up to two weeks. These are a great resource. Other overripe fruit such as peaches or berries can be frozen and used in smoothies as well. The more frozen fruit, the thicker the smoothie. Frozen fruit is preferable to ice, which will dilute your smoothie when it melts.

The following four smoothies, one for each season, are just enough for one adult, or an adult and a baby to share. Your baby will love sharing your smoothie, and this makes a fun afternoon snack together. An iced tea spoon is a good size for sharing, if neither of you has a cold, of course. Enjoy!

WINTER SMOOTHIE

$^1/_2$ *cup plain yogurt*
$^1/_2$ *cup milk*
$^1/_2$ *cup cranberry sauce, canned or homemade (recipe follows)*
1 apple, peeled, cored, and cut into big chunks
dash of cinnamon
1 frozen banana

Combine everything in a blender. Blend until smooth. Serve immediately. Serves one grown-up and one baby.

SUGAR-FREE CRANBERRY SAUCE

1 lb. fresh cranberries
1 can unsweetened apple juice concentrate
$^1/_2$ *cup orange juice concentrate*
$^1/_2$ *cup water*
$^1/_4$ *teaspoon cinnamon*

Combine first four ingredients in a medium saucepan. Bring to a boil, skim the foam, lower heat, and simmer for 15 minutes (cranberries should pop open). Remove from heat, press through a sieve or colander to remove the skins, and stir in cinnamon. This sauce is a beautiful, opaque, ruby color. It doesn't gel like cranberry sauce with sugar, but it is great to add to yogurt, applesauce, ice cream, or smoothies, and it freezes well, too.

Spring Smoothie

¹/₂ cup plain yogurt
¹/₂ cup milk
1 4-oz. can crushed pineapple
2 kiwi fruits, peeled and sliced
¹/₄ cup orange juice concentrate
1 frozen banana

Combine in a blender. Blend until smooth. Serve immediately. Serves one grown-up and one baby.

Summer Smoothie

¹/₂ cup plain yogurt
¹/₂ cup milk
1 large ripe peach or nectarine, cut into chunks
10 fresh or frozen strawberries, halved
2 tablespoons frozen orange juice concentrate
1 frozen banana

Combine in a blender. Blend until smooth. Serve immediately. Serves one grown-up and one baby.

Autumn Smoothie

¹/₂ cup plain yogurt
¹/₂ cup plain milk
¹/₄ cup canned pumpkin
¹/₄ cup unsweetened applesauce
¹/₂ teaspoon cinnamon
¹/₄ teaspoon nutmeg
dash of ginger
1 frozen banana

Combine in a blender. Blend until smooth. Serve immediately. Serves one grown-up and one baby.

Painless Ways for Breastfeeding Mothers to Get Enough Calcium

Even if you don't care for milk, there are many delicious, low-fat ways to sneak calcium into your diet. Milk is easily disguised. Also, vegans (strict vegetarians who don't consume any animal products, including dairy products) may use the calcium from vegetable sources more efficiently than milk drinkers. The following snacks and meals are so delicious, you might keep on eating them and serving them to your family long after you have weaned your baby.

- *Crunchy Broccoli.* Steam broccoli florets, then toss with Parmesan cheese and sesame seeds. Serve hot. Delicious!

- *Hearty Breakfast Skillet.* Beat 4 eggs, and combine with 1 10-or 16-ounce block mashed firm tofu, 1 cup chopped broccoli, and a corn tortilla cut into short strips. Fry in a skillet with a small amount of butter or nonstick cooking spray. When eggs are no longer wet, add $1/2$ cup to 1 cup shredded Swiss or cheddar cheese and $1/2$ cup cottage cheese. Toss until hard cheese starts to melt. Serve immediately (and soak the pan immediately, too). Serves four, including a hungry toddler (six if you use the 16-ounce tofu).

- *Cottage Cheese Dessert.* This dessert is good in the winter when fresh fruit is hard to find because canned fruit works just as well. With an ice cream scoop, scoop a mound of cottage cheese into a sundae glass, goblet, or other attractive dish. Top with your favorite chopped fruit (pineapple, banana, mandarin oranges, apricots, and peaches are all good), chopped almonds (also calcium-rich), a sprinkle of cinnamon, and a drizzle of calcium-added orange juice. (For a special treat, a little chocolate syrup is good, too!)

◉ *Collards and Beans.* Steam frozen collard greens (easier to prepare than fresh when you are pressed for time or energy) and mix $\frac{1}{2}$ cup greens with $\frac{1}{2}$ cup canned, well-rinsed white beans. Sprinkle with sesame seeds.

Meals for the Fledgling Feeder and Family

When your baby first begins solids, try foods one at a time, a week apart. When you know your baby tolerates certain foods—say, applesauce and sweet potatoes—then you can mix them together.

A Puree Rainbow

Any or all of the following fruits and vegetables can be made into a smooth puree, for use as a first food for the baby and a nutritious sauce for the rest of the family. Make a large batch of whatever vegetable or fruit is in season. Buy in bulk. Serve some of what you make that day, then freeze the rest in ice cube trays. Later, pop out the cubes and store in freezer bags, labeled and dated. One to four cubes are easily

The Basics of Homemade Baby Food

Everything must be clean. Infants are more susceptible to bacteria than adults, whose systems are stronger and more mature. Therefore, be sure that all your pots, pans, spoons, spatulas, mixing bowls, ice cube trays, cups, baby spoons, and hands are clean whenever your baby's food is touching them. Antibacterial soap is great to have at all your sinks.

Waste not, want not. Whenever you make a batch of food, immediately put aside what you will eat for that meal, then pour the rest into ice cube trays, freezer bags, or freezer containers. Label, date, and freeze. Then, on days when you really don't have time to make a meal, you can be assured that your freezer is well stocked and ready. Be sure to freeze food right away. Food left out can spoil quickly.

Taste everything first. If your baby has to eat it, you should be able to eat it. If anything has spoiled, better you discover it than your baby. Also, if anything is too hot, too cold, or too spicy, you'll know it before you spoon it into your baby's mouth. However, just because you don't like the taste of something, or if it seems to need more salt, sugar, spices, or flavor, don't assume your baby won't like it. He doesn't share your sophisticated palate (yet!) or your taste for added flavorings and sweeteners.

removed and defrosted for the baby. Breastmilk and, when your doctor says it's O.K., whole milk can be mixed with any of the defrosted cubes to make the taste more familiar or the texture creamier.

Cubes can also be removed and defrosted for the family, for use as a sauce on meat, poultry, fish, vegetables, potatoes, pancakes, yogurt, ice cream, or whatever else strikes your fancy.

Defrosting several cubes of contrasting colors—for example carrots and broccoli or peaches and pears—then swirling them atop mashed potatoes or a bowl of yogurt, or just eating them alone, makes a fun, healthy, and beautiful Puree Rainbow.

Fruits and Vegetables for Your Puree Rainbow

carrots
sweet potatoes
butternut and acorn
  squash
beets
green beans
zucchini
potatoes (puree with
  breastmilk or whole
  milk)
broccoli
peas

apples
cantaloupe
pears
peaches
nectarines
apricots
plums
prunes
dried apricots
raisins

Note: One cup of any dried fruits simmered with one can of unsweetened apple juice concentrate and pureed makes a delicious, sweet, sugar-free spread for toast, pancakes, biscuits, or cake.

Choose a vegetable or fruit. Wash, peel, cut into large pieces, and put in a saucepan. Barely cover with pure water, apple juice, or white grape juice. Bring to a low boil, then simmer, covered, for 20 minutes or until very soft. Watch carefully and add more

ENRICH YOUR LIFE

Most babies love applesauce and plain yogurt. Unsweetened applesauce, though not unhealthy, doesn't contain many vitamins (read the label). Yogurt is high in calcium and protein, but can also be enriched.

Add some of any of the following (anywhere from 2 tablespoons to $1/4$ cup) to 1 cup of applesauce or plain yogurt. Whatever your baby doesn't finish, you can eat. (It would be a shame to waste such good food.) All combinations are delicious and good for you.

- canned pumpkin (high in beta carotene)

- cranberry sauce (high in vitamin C—see page 253 for a homemade, sugarless recipe)

- 1 or 2 cubes of frozen fruit or vegetable puree, defrosted

- wheat germ

- mashed banana

- orange juice concentrate

- apple juice concentrate (find the kind with added vitamin C)

water or juice if necessary, but boil with as little liquid as possible, to avoid discarding vitamins. Alternatively, you can steam any produce in a steamer basket, which preserves more vitamins.

When the fruit or vegetable is soft, cool slightly and transfer to a blender. Don't fill the blender more than halfway; it may splatter. Include just enough cooking juice to make blending easy. Puree on high speed until smooth. If desired, especially for younger babies, strain the mixture through a sieve or cheesecloth. Set aside enough for the day's meal, and refrigerate. Pour the remaining puree into ice cube trays. Freeze and store as directed above.

When your baby is a little older, try out the following delicious puree combinations. Blend thoroughly, or swirl for a marbled effect:

> *apples and sweet potatoes*
> *broccoli and butternut or acorn squash*
> *peaches and pears*
> *apples and pears*
> *carrots and butternut or acorn squash*
> *beets and white potatoes*
> *peaches and plums*
> *any combination of the dried fruits*

Autumn Harvest Soup

> *2 medium sweet potatoes (about 1 lb.)*
> *1 lb. carrots*
> *4 cups vegetable or chicken broth (homemade or low-sodium canned)*
> *1 12-oz. can apple juice concentrate*
> *1 teaspoon cinnamon*
> *1/2 teaspoon nutmeg*
> *1/2 teaspoon ginger*
> *2 cups skim milk*
> *2 tablespoons breastmilk (or spring water)*
> *1/2 cup pecans, chopped and toasted*

Wash the sweet potatoes, prick, and bake in the oven (about 1 hour at 400 degrees) or microwave (about 11 minutes on high for two medium potatoes) until soft. Cut potatoes open and scrape insides with a spoon into a small bowl. Set aside. While sweet potatoes are cooking, wash and scrape the carrots, cutting off ends. Cut into 2-inch pieces. In a large pot, combine carrot pieces, broth, and apple juice concentrate. Bring to a boil, lower heat, cover, and simmer for 20 minutes. Remove pot from heat. With a slotted spoon, transfer carrot pieces to a blender, along with $\frac{1}{2}$ cup to 1 cup liquid. Puree on high until smooth.

Remove $\frac{1}{2}$ cup carrot puree to a small bowl, combine with $\frac{1}{2}$ cup of the sweet potatoes, and set aside (for the baby).

Return the remaining puree to the pan. Add remaining sweet potatoes to the pot. Add spices and stir to combine. Return to a simmer. Cook, stirring occasionally, for 15 minutes.

While soup is simmering, press carrot-potato mixture you have set aside through a sieve or cheesecloth, if desired. Stir in breastmilk or water. Set aside for the baby.

Remove soup from heat and stir in skim milk. Ladle into bowls for the rest of the family. Garnish each bowl with toasted pecans (none for the baby yet, of course).

Serves eight (or four as a main course) plus a baby.

FAMILY DINNERS FOR THE SIX- TO EIGHT-MONTH-OLD

At this age, your baby can handle more interesting combinations of food. Now is the time to experiment with puree mixtures and coarser textures (blend on low instead of high). A baby can also handle soft finger food cut into small pieces.

Sunday Chicken (or Butternut) Dinner

1 fryer chicken (3 to 5 lbs.) or 1 large or 2 medium
  butternut squashes, peeled and cubed into large dice
6 cups water
1 large yellow onion
3 carrots, peeled and sliced into 2-inch pieces
3 celery stalks, sliced into 2-inch pieces
5 cloves garlic, peeled and halved
10 white mushrooms, halved
1/2 medium turnip, peeled and cut into large dice
small handful fresh parsley
1 teaspoon dried sage
1 teaspoon dried thyme
4 medium baking potatoes
1 cup sour cream (low-or nonfat is delicious)
black pepper, freshly grated
1/2 cup shredded cheddar or mozzarella cheese
  (optional)

Combine the first eleven ingredients in a large pot or Dutch oven. Bring to a boil, lower heat, skim any foam, cover, and simmer for 2 hours, stirring occasionally. If you are using the squash, don't add it until the second hour.

Meanwhile, scrub potatoes, prick, and put in a preheated 400-degree oven for 1 hour (or bake in the microwave on high, arranging potatoes like spokes of a wheel, for 20 minutes).

Remove pot from heat. Put a colander over a large bowl in the sink. Remove chicken (it will probably fall apart, but get the

FATHER ALERT!

EASY ROMANCE

Now that baby makes three (or more if you have other kids), you will want to take every opportunity for some romantic time alone with your wife. Treat her one evening, after the baby is asleep, to this simple and elegant picnic supper, preferably spread out on a tablecloth on the living room floor. Candlelight adds a nice ambiance.

◎ Buy a loaf of really good, fresh French or Italian bread from the bakery.

◎ Buy a good-quality, mild, soft cheese such as Brie, Camembert, Havarti, Muenster, or Fontina.

◎ Make an antipasto (Italian for "appetizer") plate by arranging any combination of the following on a nice platter or tray (make it look artistic—this is your chance to show your creativity!)

> *olives*
> *pepperoncini*
> *marinated artichoke hearts*
> *slices of turkey pastrami or other deli meat, rolled*
> *   up and secured with a toothpick*
> *tiny pickles*
> *baby carrots*
> *radishes*
> *a vine-ripened tomato, sliced*
> *fresh grapes*
> *a Granny Smith apple, cored, sliced, and rubbed*
> *   with a cut lemon to prevent browning*
> *strawberries or other good, fresh berries*

Serve the bread, cheese, and antipasto platter on nice dishes with sparkling red or white grape juice in champagne glasses. Talk, and focus on each other. If your baby does wake up, don't let him spoil the party. Instead, let him join you. He'll probably enjoy looking at the candles, and they may even lull him back to sleep. The point is to have a nice, relaxing meal and enjoy each other's company again.

biggest pieces) to the colander and allow the stock to drain into the bowl. Then carefully pull off as much of the meat as you can and set aside. Discard the bones.

Pour the remaining contents of the pot into the colander. Remove most of the remaining meat to the plate. Discard all remaining bones. (You may have to wait until it all cools down.)

If you are using the squash, simply pour the entire pot into the colander to drain off the stock, then separate out the cubes of squash from the other vegetables and set aside.

One or two cups at a time, put cooked vegetables into a blender with a small amount of stock. Puree and pour into a bowl. Reserve remaining stock for another use (freeze it in ice cube trays for future blending uses or a quick soup base).

Slice open each potato and scoop out pulp with a spoon into a mixing bowl. Add the sour cream and beat on low speed until creamy and smooth.

For the baby, combine $1/2$ cup mashed potatoes with vegetable puree and 1 tablespoon of the optional shredded cheese.

For the rest of the family, divide the remaining potatoes between three or four plates, forming a well in the center of each potato mound. Top each with chunks of chicken or cubes of squash. Pour vegetable puree over the top as a sauce. Top with pepper and garnish with shredded cheese, if desired. Serves four plus a baby.

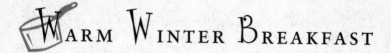Warm Winter Breakfast

2 cups cooked brown rice (a good way to use leftover rice)
1 cup whole milk
1/4 cup nonfat dry milk
1/4 cup wheat germ
1/4 cup frozen orange juice concentrate
1/2 cup finely chopped dried apricots and/or raisins

Combine all ingredients in a large saucepan. Slowly heat to a low simmer, stirring frequently. Do not boil. Serves three to four plus a baby.

If you are up for a mess, put this in a bowl for the baby and let her try to eat it with a spoon and/or her hands.

Family Meals for the Eight- to Twelve-month-old Baby

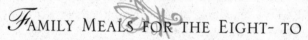Quick And Light Italian Supper

This recipe uses several canned ingredients, some high in salt. However, most of the salty ingredients aren't in the baby's serving. Feel free to omit the artichokes or olives if you don't like them. It will still work.

¹/₂ lb. three-color rotini pasta
1 16-oz. can whole tomatoes
2 large cloves garlic, peeled and quartered
¹/₂ cup Parmesan cheese
1 4-oz. can sliced black olives, drained and rinsed well
1 4-oz. can marinated artichoke hearts, undrained
1 can white beans, drained and rinsed well
Optional accompaniments: salad, fresh bread

Boil the rotini according to package directions. Drain and rinse. (You might want to cook your baby's portion a little longer if you prefer yours *al dente*.)

In a blender, combine the canned tomatoes, garlic, and Parmesan cheese. Blend until garlic is chopped and sauce appears smooth. Pour out ½ cup into your baby's bowl, then pour the remaining mixture into a saucepan (or the warm pasta pot). Add the drained olives and the undrained artichoke hearts with liquid. Put ½ cup of the beans into your baby's bowl, then add the remaining beans to the sauce. Stir and heat through.

For the baby, toss ½ cup rotini (you might want to cut each twist in half for easier handling) with the beans and sauce, and let the baby go at it!

For the rest of the family, ladle the warm sauce over bowls of rotini.

Serve with a salad and fresh bread, if desired. (Give your baby cubes of bread, too, if you serve it. Wait on the lettuce.) Serves four plus a baby.

GREAT FINGER FOODS

Make sure everything is cut to size until your baby has figured out how to bite off small pieces.

- canned beans (white, red, pinto, black, etc.), drained and well rinsed (to remove excess salt)

- cubes of whole wheat bread or toast (with or without butter and/or fruit spread)

- scrambled eggs or an omelet cut in strips (yolks only, until your doctor says whites are O.K.)

- stubby, well-cooked pasta (whole wheat is best, but white, spinach, tomato, and other flavors are a nice change, if your baby likes them)

- brown rice

- peeled, chopped, fresh tomatoes

- sliced banana (the riper it is, the more digestible)

- cottage cheese (low sodium is best)

- small cubes or shreds of mozzarella, cheddar, or Swiss cheese (low sodium, if you can find it)

- slightly mashed, well-cooked peas

- cubed white and sweet potatoes

- well-cooked broccoli florets

- well-cooked green beans (remove the strings)

- canned, crushed pineapple (or chunk, but cut the chunks into fourths if they are too big)

- round oat cereal

- cubed, whole-grain pumpkin muffins
- chicken, turkey, white fish, beef, or lamb, well cooked and chopped into small pieces
- cubed, very ripe peaches, pears, plums, melons, kiwi, mangoes, etc. (any soft fruit)
- soft, well-cooked cubes of carrots and the winter squashes
- tiny meatballs (try ground turkey)
- cubes of soft tofu

BROCCOLI CHEESE POTATOES

4 potatoes, baked
2 cups broccoli, cooked soft
1 cup cooked brown rice
1/4 cup Parmesan cheese
1/2 cup to 1 cup water or vegetable stock (canned or homemade)

Skin and cube the smallest potato. Put into your baby's bowl.

Combine broccoli, brown rice, Parmesan cheese, and a small amount of stock or water in the blender. Puree until smooth. Add more water if necessary.

Toss 1/2 cup puree with cubed potatoes in the baby's bowl. Serve as finger food.

Top the remaining three potatoes with the broccoli-cheese sauce. Freeze any remaining sauce in ice cube trays for future use. The sauce is a great baby food on its own, too. Serves three plus a baby.

Enjoy

Once you've become more comfortable with cooking for your baby, new ideas for recipes, finger foods, and smoothie combinations will occur to you. Don't be afraid to experiment. The baby who is used to trying a variety of foods will be a healthier eater and, perhaps someday, a fantastic and innovative cook.

☙ · RESOURCES

Take a look at the following listings of organizations and web sites on breastfeeding, parenting, nutrition, the workplace, and more for great tips, information, and advice.

The American Academy of Pediatrics
141 Northwest Point Boulevard
Elk Grove Village, IL 60007-1098
Phone: (847) 228-5005
Web site: *www.aap.org*
Keep up with the latest in the field of pediatrics.

American College of Obstetricians and Gynecologists
409 12th Street, SW
PO Box 96920
Washington, DC 20090-8920
Phone: (202) 638-5577
Web site: *www.acog.org*

American Dietetic Association
216 West Jackson Boulevard, Suite 800
Chicago, IL 60606-6995
Phone: (800) 877-1600
Web site: *www.eatright.org*
The ADA and its National Center for Nutrition and Dietetics promote optimal nutrition, health, and well-being.

Best Start
3500 East Fletcher Avenue, Suite 519
Tampa, FL 33613
Phone: (800) 277-4975
Promotes breastfeeding for the economically disadvantaged.

Cybermom
Web site: *www.thecyber-mom.com*

A great on-line magazine "for Moms with Modems."

Families and Work Institute
330 Seventh Avenue
New York, NY 10001
Phone: (212) 465-2044
Web site: *www.familiesand-workinst.org*
The institute identifies and studies emerging work-life trends and issues, considering the entire life cycle, from prenatal and child care to elder care.

Food Co-ops
Web site:
www.columbia.edu/-jw15-7/food.coop.html#resources
A listing of organic food coops across the country. Look for one in your area.

Go Organic Online
Web site: *www.go-organic.com*
A place to learn about organic products, discuss issues relating to organic foods, and buy organic products in the Internet Green Marketplace®.

International Lactation Consultant Association
4101 Lake Boone Trail
Raleigh, NC 27607
Phone: (919) 787-5181
Web site: *www.ilca.org*
The ILCA promotes the professional development, advancement, and recognition of lactation consultants worldwide for breastfeeding women, infants, and children.

KidsHealth.Org
Web site: *www.kidshealth.org*
Medical experts at the Alfred I. DuPont Hospital for Children, the Nemours Children's Clinics and other children's health facilities nationwide contribute information on children's health topics.

Interactive Pregnancy Calendar
Web site: *www.pregnancycalendar.com*
If you're even considering another pregnancy, check out this fun site, which creates a personalized pregnancy calendar, or even a personalized ovulation calendar, just for you.

LaLeche League International
1400 N. Meacham Road
Schaumburg, IL
60173-4048
Phone: (847)-7730
Web site: *www.laleche-league.org*
An organization solely devoted to breastfeeding. The web site includes many links to other relevant Internet resources.

Medscape
Web site:
www.medscape.com
A comprehensive health information web site.

National Association for Family Child Care
1331A Pennsylvania Avenue NW, Suite 348
Washington, DC 20004
Phone: (800) 359-3817 (Child care)
(800) 628-9163 (Day care)
A clearinghouse for child care issues.

National Foundation for Women Business Owners
1100 Wayne Ave., Suite 830
Silver Spring, MD
20910-5603

Phone: (301) 495-4975
Web site: *www.nfwbo.org*
Affiliated with the National Association of Women Business Owners, this organization promotes the entrepreneurial interests of women.

National Institutes of Health
National Institute of Child Health and Human Development
Web site: *www.nih.gov*
Research in all health fields, and particular research at NICHHD on children's health topics.

National Women's Health Network
514 10th St. NW, Suite 400
Washington, DC 20005
Phone: (202)347-1140
A leading health advocacy organization on women's health issues, and a great source of information.

Open-Air Market Net
Web site: *www.openair.org*
A worldwide guide to farmers' markets, street markets, and other markets. Check for resources in your area.

ParentsPlace
Web site:
  www.parentsplace.com
Everything and more for new
parents. Get a free weekly
newsletter.

ParentSoup
Web site:
  www.parentsoup.com
Another great general-interest
web site for parents.

Parents Without Partners
401 North Michigan Avenue
Chicago, IL 60611-4267
Phone: (800) 637-7974
A self-help organization with
resources for divorced, wid-
owed, or never-married parents.

Single Mothers by Choice
P.O. Box 1642
New York, NY 10028
Phone: (212) 988-0993
Web site:
  *www.parentsplace.com/
  read-room/smc*

A national organization for
single women who are con-
sidering becoming, or who
have become, mothers by
choice. A great organization
to approach for support and
advice.

Vegetarian Pages
Web site:
  www.veg.org/veg
A comprehensive guide to
vegetarian resources on the
Internet.

Veggies Unite!
PO Box 5312
Fort Wayne, IN
  46895-5312
Web site:
  www.vegweb.com
A great source for vegetarian
recipes, with weekly meal
planning, conversion tables,
and other interactive stuff,
including more recipes
than you could ever
prepare.

❧· Suggested Reading

About Breastfeeding

Eiger, Marvin S. and Sally Wendkos Olds. *The Complete Book of Breastfeeding*. New York: Workman Publishing, 1987.

Gotsch, Gwen and La Leche International. *Breastfeeding Pure and Simple*. Franklin Park, Illinois: La Leche League International, 1994.

Gotsch, Gwen, Judy Torgus and La Leche International. *The Womanly Art of Breastfeeding*. Franklin Park, Illinois: La Leche International, 1997.

Grame, Marilyn. *Breastfeeding Source Book: Where to Get What You Need to Breastfeed Successfully*. Sheridan, Wyoming: Achievement Press, 1988.

About Baby Care, Parenting, and Family

Elium, Jean and Don Elium. *Raising a Daughter: Parents and the Awakening of a Healthy Woman*. Berkeley, California: Celestial Arts, 1994.

———. *Raising a Son: Parents and the Awakening of a Healthy Man*. Berkeley, California: Celestial Arts, 1996.

276 · *Suggested Reading*

Eisenberg, Arlene, Heidi E. Murkoff, and Sandee E. Hathaway. *What to Expect the First Year*. New York: Workman Publishing, 1994.

———. *What to Expect When You're Expecting*. London: Simon and Schuster, 1993.

Sears, William and Martha Sears. *The Baby Book*. Boston and London: Little, Brown and Co., 1993.

Sears, William. *Creative Parenting: How to Use the New Continuum Concept to Raise Children Successfully from Birth to Adolescence*. New York: Everest House, 1982.

———. *Nighttime Parenting: How to Get Your Baby to Sleep*. New York: New American Library, 1987.

Shelov, Steven, editor, et. al. The American Academy of Pediatrics *Caring for Your Baby and Young Child, Birth to Age 5*. New York: Bantam Books, 1993.

About Nutrition and Cooking

Better Homes and Gardens New Cookbook. New York: Bantam Books, 1993.

Diamond, Marilyn. *The American Vegetarian Cookbook: From the Fit for Life Kitchen*. New York: Warner Books, 1990.

Eshleman, Ruthe. *The American Heart Association Cookbook*. New York: D. McKay Co., 1973.

Katzen, Mollie. *Moosewood Cookbook*. Berkeley, California: Ten Speed Press, 1992.

Lansky, Vicki. *Fat-Proofing Your Child—So They Don't Become Diet Addicted Adults*. Toronto and New York: Bantam Books, 1988.

———. *Feed Me! I'm Yours: Delicious, Nutritious, and Fun Things to Cook Up for Your Kids*. Deephaven, Minnesota: Meadowbrook Press, 1984.

Thomas, Anna. *New Vegetarian Epicure*. New York: Viking Penguin, 1991.

Rosso, Julee. *Fresh Start: Great Low-Fat Recipes, Day-by-Day Menus—The Savvy Way to Cook, Eat, and Live*. New York: Crown Publishers, 1996.

About Health Care

Balch, James F. and Phyllis A. Balch. *Prescription for Nutritional Healing*. Garden City Park, New York: Avery Publishing Group, Inc., 1990.

Kastner, Mark and Hugh Burroughs. *Alternative Healing: The Complete A–Z Guide to Over 160 Different Alternative Therapies*. La Mesa, California: Halcyon Publishing, 1993.

Mayell Mark and the Editors of Natural Health Magazine. *52 Simple Steps to Natural Health: A Week-by-Week Guide to More Healthful Living*. New York: Pocket Books, 1995.

Olkin, Sylvia Klein. *Positive Parenting Fitness: A Parent's Resource Guide to Nutrition, Stress Reduction, Total Exercise and Practical Information*. Garden City Park, New York: Avery Publishing Group, Inc., 1997.